My Father Forgets

12-14-90

Kathy—I know this is
an odd birthday present—
But has our friendship ever
been anything but odd?
May it always remain
just so—

Love—
Eileen

My Father Forgets

By
Lynn McAndrews

NORTHERN PUBLISHING
Maple City, Michigan

Additional copies of this book may be ordered through bookstores or by sending $8.95 plus $2.50 for postage and handling to Northern Publishing, P.O. Box 136, Maple City, MI 49664

A portion of the profits from the sale of this book will be donated to the Alzheimer's Disease and Related Disorders Association for research into the cause and treatment of Alzheimer's disease

Published by
Northern Publishing
Post Office Box 136
Maple City, Michigan 49664

LIBRARY OF CONGRESS
CATALOG CARD NUMBER: 90-091658
ISBN #0-9626683-0-3

Dedicated to my mother, Viola Dechow,
and to all caregivers, mostly women,
who give of themselves for dementia victims.

Table of Contents

Preface

Dear Reader,

I share this book with you not to frighten you or ask for your sympathy. Rather, my goal is to offer some insight into the devastation that Alzheimer's disease causes its victims and families. With insight, I hope that you might be better prepared should this happen to one you love. May you also be more understanding should one of your friends or neighbors suffer from this disease.

I have discovered through my work with the hospice movement that we find it difficult to talk openly about dying. Many books have now been written about grief, bereavement, and dying. But we still struggle to openly express our thoughts and feelings.

I have not downplayed the sadness and difficulties that my family experienced. I use the words death and dying freely and I describe the stages of the disease in detail. Some may find this approach "depressing." I believe it is the disease that is depressing, not the manner of the telling.

We take what life gives us and do the best that we can, and that is what our family did as we watched my father die. The sharing of emotions that we experienced and the actions that we took may help you to know that you are not alone. If you are a professional working with dementia victims and their families, reading this account may give you insight into a family's side of the story.

Many thanks to all of those who shared their part of the story, especially members of my family, Darlene and John, Jon and Esther, Paul and Joanne, Jim, and Mother.

My hope is that you will be moved to donate your time and money to groups dedicated to fighting this dread disease. Years from now may we look back and find Alzheimer's disease only a memory.

Lynn McAndrews
May 1990

Introduction

Death, disease, and the aging process are facts of life and of nature. In spite of this, the prevailing American attitude toward these phenomena is that of denial. Most of us in today's youth-obsessed society prefer not to think about such unpleasant topics until the events of life take over and we are forced to deal with these distressing forms of loss. It is then that we are likely to find ourselves unprepared to face the ordeal of learning to care for a loved one in decline.

In our culture we are allowed to grow well into adulthood largely protected from the problems encountered by the aging and, in particular, diseases mostly associated with aging. No longer living in extended families, we remain unaware of the daily, gradual changes experienced by even the healthiest of our elders. As a society we demonstrate little appreciation for the challenges these processes present.

The following pages illustrate that the effects of Alzheimer's on everyone involved can be dramatic and devastating. Faced with any disease that robs one of the use of one's body, or undermines one's sense of self through disorientation and lapses of memory, both the victim and his or her loved ones suffer a painful and frightening loss. Compounding that loss, unfortunately, may be a lack of understanding, resulting partly from our tendency to avoid this disturbing subject matter until the need to deal with it intrudes on our lives.

In writing of her father's, and indeed her entire family's, experience with Alzheimer's, Lynn McAndrews offers us the opportunity to increase our understanding of a reality which could touch the lives of any of us. Her intimate portrayal of the events leading up to her father's death invokes our compassion and sharpens our appreciation for the simplest of human interactions. We see, as the disease advances, that his sense of identity becomes increasingly fragile, and so does his ability to respond to those who know and love him. Thus, in a style more direct than sentimental, McAndrews widens our perspective on what truly matters in life, not by spelling it out, but more through what is gracefully left unsaid.

My Father Forgets is a gift to us of compassion and empathy for a generation too often ignored and of which we will all, in our turn, become members. This very moving and human story gently reminds us of — and prepares us to face — one of nature's "sweet sorrows"; namely, that loss is a fact of life and, especially, of love.

Camille Vettraino
May 15, 1990

My Father Forgets

Chapter I - Death

On the eve of Palm Sunday my father starved to death. In his last months his body became weak and frail, 85 pounds of skin and bones. His communication had dwindled to a blank stare. He had no control over his body. Sometimes he would soil his pants and need his diaper changed like a newborn baby. Mental processes, too, seemed to have stopped. Yet I wanted to believe he recognized my mother and me sitting at his death bed.

His gaze was piercing, but his awareness was rapidly failing in his last hours. Nevertheless I feel he knew we were there. His supposed awareness was one small thing I could cling to, knowing that he had endured the erosion of his pride and dignity, the loss of his mind, and that he was dying.

The pale skin shone through the thin white hair lying limply on his rounded head. His still form lay under the blanket as if nothing were there. Occasionally his legs contorted into a rigid posture and only returned to a lying position when assisted. His skin was still warm to the touch, offsetting the pallor it exhibited to the eye.

As I sat there holding his hand, I remembered a better time. In my mind's eye I saw a man wearing a well tailored brown tweed suit, whose face was clean shaven, hair slicked back and combed neatly. I smelled the Old Spice cologne he used to wear. I saw him talking gregariously with a few church members after the service and then I heard him chuckle, shaking his head back and forth and clucking his tongue, the way he used to when something amused him.

I remembered riding to high school with him one warm spring day when he shared with me that although he had had opportunities, he had never been unfaithful to my mother. I wasn't sure why he told me that, but now I understand he was trying to teach me about the future temptations I might face.

I recalled the onion poultice (an old sock full of cooked onions and hot water) that he used to put around my neck when I had a chest cold. I hated the smell, but loved the attention.

I felt the silence as our family drove from the church to the cemetery after my uncle's funeral. I saw my father cry at the loss of his brother and knew that this was one of the few times he would allow himself that type of release for his pain.

I remembered the way he cocked his head to one side and smiled sweetly when he called me his "Mame Doll." I felt embarrassed, but pleased, when he used that endearing term. I longed to hear it once more. I wanted to see him one more time walking from the house to the garden unassisted, getting the tools from the garage to work on the weeds that needed attention. I wanted to go back and see him and my mother go out for yet one more square dance, him in his western outfit and her with her full skirt and petticoat, on their way to have fun.

No death is easy to watch, but his I imagined to be worse than most. He did not seem in physical pain. Yet, since he was unable to communicate, there was no way we could ever really know the extent of his suffering.

Many diseases have physical suffering of greater intensity, but the gradual loss of one's mental faculties over the course of five to fifteen years is an ordeal no one should have to endure. The illness's effect on its victim can only be left to the imagination of those who must watch and wait. I thought of the times he must have been aware of what was happening to his memory and hoped his recognition had not lasted long. Painkillers are available for physical pain. What is there for the mental anguish of memory loss and dementia?

My father's disease progressed faster than other cases. Yet my mother, who was the one who lived with him day in and day out and knew of his personality changes, argues that he had had Alzheimer's longer than the rest of the family realized.

He starved to death, literally. Alzheimer's patients never really die from the disease, but from complications, such as pneumonia. Our family decided not to prolong Dad's dying through artificial life support systems and, thus, we did not move him to a hospital from the nursing home. So he starved to death, because the disease's final assault on him, as on most, took away his ability to swallow.

He forgot his loved ones' faces, names, any association at all with them. He could not remember anything from one minute to the next, how and when to urinate and defecate, how to eat, walk, and talk. Finally, his brain forgot how to tell his muscles to swallow. Nurses, their aides, social workers, and loved ones helped him walk and go to the bathroom; they even changed his diapers; but they couldn't help him swallow. Suction was used to clear the throat, and then some liquid would make its way down to quench his thirst, but in the end the muscles constricted and would not allow passage.

I remember the last day vividly. It was a cool Saturday spring morning, April 14, 1984. Though clouds were threatening to sprinkle rain, the winter's snow had been melting and the hope of warmer weather was in the air. After briefly inspecting the goods at a local farm auction that morning, my mother and I had gone to the nursing home to see how my father was doing.

We knew he was getting worse and could die at any time, but we were not prepared for the nurse's announcement when we arrived at the nursing home about 11:30 a.m. In response to my comment that his condition appeared worse, she said, "Yes. I was going to call you."

"Why were you going to call us?" I asked.

"Oh, to find out where to send him."

At first I thought she meant which hospital. Then I realized she was talking about which funeral home. *"A rather abrupt way of putting it,"* I thought. The nurse told us that death could come at any time now, in a few days or a few hours.

Having inherited my father's aptitude for organization, I went into action. My mother and I quickly discussed the possibility of requesting an autopsy. Since this is the only sure way to know if he had Alzheimer's, we decided to have one. We had discussed it before, and I had thought about it myself too. I knew the only part necessary to be analyzed was the brain. Its removal would have no effect upon an open casket funeral, which is what both parents had wanted. I wanted the nagging doubts and questions erased from my mind. Death raises enough questions on its own. We could control the answer to one of those questions. In addition, I had heard that the brains of Alzheimers' patients were needed to assist in research toward finding its cure and that of other illnesses.

I called one of the local hospitals and talked to a pathologist. He was unaware of who would pay what for this procedure, but said he would contact the University of Michigan where local brains needing autopsy were sent, and he would see what arrangements could be made. He promised to return my call.

All of this was done out of earshot of my father. He seemed totally unaware, but I knew that one of the last senses to be lost was hearing. I remembered horror stories of people surviving a near death and speaking of how they had heard others in the room planning their funerals before they were even gone.

In my father's case it wasn't really necessary to plan the funeral, because he had done just about everything imaginable beforehand — several years earlier, in fact. John Theodor Dechow had been a person who had always planned ahead and took his family responsibilities very seriously. He had his funeral details arranged even to the Scripture passage and hymns to be used. Romans 10:9, my father's favorite passage, was the one he had chosen: "If thou shalt confess with thy mouth the Lord Jesus, and shalt believe in thine heart that God hath raised him from the dead, thou shalt be saved." He had recited the verse to my younger brother Paul and I whenever he was afraid we had strayed from the faith.

Standing there at the nurses' station as people walked in and out, I was talking to the funeral director and the pathologist and making arrangements for my father's demise. He was only two doors away, still alive, unaware of my following in his footsteps by being organized and planning ahead. I had learned my lessons well from him. It still amazes me what a human being is capable of doing when faced with an urgent need such as the imminent loss of one's parent.

The pathologist called back shortly and said there would be no charge from the University of Michigan for the autopsy, since donations of brains were needed for research. That was a relief. I had heard the cost could be six to eight hundred dollars. However, he said he would have to charge $100 for removal of the brain from the body and transporting it to the university. And of course, they would need to act quickly, and the funeral home would have to know about this so that the body could be transported to the hospital before embalming.

I notified the funeral director, whom my family had known for years, of these decisions. We also decided that if anyone could use my father's eyes we would donate them. I notified the hospital about this, too. We discovered later that no one had removed them because he was "too old."

After the necessary phone calls, I went back into my father's room where my mother was sitting with him. Appearing much younger than her 68 years, she was a pretty woman. Just the same, the stress of his illness had left her physically and mentally exhausted. She sat quietly at his bedside, holding his hand, gazing first at his face, then down at the floor, then out the window. His eyes were open and he would look at each of us, but no words came from his mouth. We wanted to believe he knew us, although there were no clear signs of recognition. We didn't know for certain that he would die today, but we knew death would be soon. Had we not been present then, I at least would have felt robbed of the comfort of knowing I had been with him to the last.

Although I had known people who were dying, I had never actually been present at a death and I honestly wondered what it would be like. I also wanted to share the experience with my mother, both for me and for her, so she would not have to be alone. I wanted my father's suffering to be over, and I hoped my presence would be comforting.

By now it was about 1:00 p.m. I had called my husband Jim and a family friend, Ron, in case they wanted to see him once more before he died. I told them his death could be at any moment. They both came in for a brief time to say goodbye.

I decided to leave the nursing home for a few hours to play in a tennis tournament to which I was committed. I had mixed feelings about doing so, but at the time I didn't know that this was my father's last day, and I honestly needed a break from his dying for a few hours. I don't regret the decision to play, nor did I experience guilt afterward as a result. Other guilty feelings surfaced later, but for different reasons. Guilt was an integral part of my life growing up. There was something about that strict, conservative, rigid, midwestern Lutheran upbringing that made one wonder whether even breathing could be a free act with no strings attached.

Later I called my mother at the nursing home to see how things were going. She had stayed on with him since morning. She said his breathing was more shallow but there hadn't been much change. The one thing she remembers most about that day is how he looked at her from the time she got there until he died: not a stare necessarily, but as if he wanted to ask her a question and could not do so.

By now it was 5:00 o'clock. I convinced her to go home and get something to eat. Within an hour or so she had returned.

I stopped at the nursing home and sat with my father for a few minutes after Mom had gone home. There was no change in his demeanor, but his flesh was still warm and alive. I held his hand and wished his dying didn't have to be this way. I didn't know how I wanted it to be, really. If I thought about it long enough, I might come to the conclusion that this was the only way for him to die — unaware. That way he wouldn't have to experience the fear associated with the process of letting go. I went home then for a brief time to meditate and get something to eat before returning.

I returned shortly after 8:00 p.m. My mother had already been there for more than an hour. It was as if my father had waited to die until I got back, because at 8:34 p.m. he stopped breathing. It was no more dramatic than that. His misery was over. Both Mother and I were crying, and she said something like, "The strife is o'er; the victory's won." I wasn't as sure about the "victory" as she seemed to be.

He was gone. No more holding his warm, strong hand and comforting him, however difficult. No more coming to visit him on his few good days when he seemed to know us. No more having him look blankly at us while we tried to read things into his stare. No more of anything with him.

Nothing more except our memories. Those memories are strong, but they do fade as time goes by. The mind can handle the loss better when the images dim. I wouldn't want to remember everything, nor do I try. But sometimes when I least expect it, I'll find myself sobbing in the middle of a public place, such as at a movie theater or on the sidewalk, and wanting desperately to be transported to a place where no one will see me, for I want my grief to be private. But it doesn't always work that way. Grief is hard, but necessary. The process helps us move on. Sometimes it is necessary to talk, to have someone listen to the pain, the sadness, the joy of memories, and then say, "It's going to be all right." Other times I just want someone to be there with me, knowing that I will be all right, but that the grief process is something I must go through.

That was the first time I had witnessed a death firsthand. I don't know what I had expected, but the event itself, at least in the next few days, wasn't as difficult emotionally as I had anticipated. My feelings were mixed, but the overwhelming one in the next few hours was re-lief: relief that his suffering was over, that our waiting for him to die was over; the interminable waiting was over.

I called the funeral director, who was there within a half hour. We waited for him to get there before we went home. We even gathered all of my father's things, even though we could have waited until later. Before we left I touched his body again. I'm not sure why I did that — perhaps to find out what a lifeless body felt like. It was cold and rigid, hard — all warmth and life gone. The man who had been my father had long since left that body. Now even his great warmth had left his body, and touch-ing it brought no comfort.

My mother and I went to my house, knowing there was no reason to stay at the nursing home. I thought of the custom in times past of the deceased being laid out in one's home. I thought of the family dressing the person and staying with the body for a couple days before the funeral. I wondered at the great sense of completion those activities must have been for those who did so. Our com-pletion that night, or at least mine, came from calling my brothers and sister with my mother at my side and inform-ing them of my father's death.

The events of the next few days up to the funeral are somewhat blurred now, but one thing that remains in my mind is the great amount of energy I had during that period and the closeness I felt to other family members. Some of that closeness has since ebbed with the tides of human relationships, but the memory of my father's passage will not be forgotten.

Chapter II - Life

"Get in this car right now!" my father demanded. He was yelling at me from his open car window. I was sitting under a tree about 75 feet off the road with my first boyfriend, Eddie. We were only talking, but my father's rage suggested we were fornicating on the front lawn. I had taken a drive with Eddie to "The Valley," only about four blocks from our suburban home, but an area of the neighborhood reputed to be a sexual experimentation ground for many a young teenager, which I was at the time. Our date was over for that afternoon. The ride home seemed an eternity. I said little, if anything, to my father. I could not share the shame, hurt, and humiliation of the moment with anyone.

As long as I can remember, John Theodor Dechow had always been a very domineering personality. His way was the right way. Compulsive in the organization of his life, he had all his nails in the right containers, on the right shelves. If he found one out of place, he wasted no time in replacing it. Having grown up in the Depression, he had learned not to spend money foolishly, but he provided well for his family and worked hard. He was a stern taskmaster and disciplinarian and, at least until recent years, I had often been afraid of him. Later, when he was so vulnerable, the thought of being fearful of him seemed ludicrous.

Growing up under John Dechow's thumb was fraught with fear and trembling. In his eyes I suspect his rigidity was his way of gaining respect from his children, but many times his inability to see the gray in a situation left no room for healthy inquiry or discussion. I recall a time when I questioned the meaning of a Bible passage and asked him about it. I quickly learned that doubting the King James version was not something one did in John Dechow's household. He yelled at me. I went to my room and cried, and that was the end of it.

Yet he was outgoing, friendly, and giving in his way, perhaps more so as he got older. He was a complicated man. On the other side of his anger was his generosity. He bought me a movie camera and projector when I was in college for my first trip to Europe, the purchase of which I'm sure he believed to be an extravagance.

It was as if he and my mother had raised two families. In 1933 he had married Viola May Behne. They had three children in three years, one of whom died in childbirth, and then 10 years later I was born, and then my younger brother arrived 6-1/2 years after that. Darlene was the first, born in 1934, and Jon was born in 1936. I know their childhood must have been filled with more fear than mine was, but my father may have learned something along the way and become more tolerant of children when Paul and I were growing up. I came along in 1946 and Paul in 1953.

My father was a teacher and school administrator most of his life. He started out in County Normal (in Leelanau County, Michigan), an "old school" method of becoming certified to teach in Michigan. He taught and coached for many years (math, shop, basketball) in northern Michigan. Then, when I was five, we moved to the southern part of the state, where he was principal of a high school outside of Battle Creek. Although very strict, my father was an inspiring teacher. Former students of his still approach me and let me know he was the finest teacher they ever had. As I remember him, his sense of right and wrong was a great asset from a moral point of view. He always seemed to do what was "right," but in the process let flexibility go by the wayside.

I fondly remember Sundays in Battle Creek. We would go to church, then out to eat, then home. The family would be together. My father was well respected. An elder of the church, he was involved in community activities.

My mother took care of the children and the house during those years and was the calm many times in the storm. When my father would get angry at me, Mom was always there for comfort and solace, although rarely did she ever talk back to him nor did she assert herself enough for her own rights.

One day when I came home from school, Mom was mopping the living room floor and sobbing, her shoulders heaving with deep sighs. He had come home angry, yelled at her for no apparent reason, then stormed out of the house. I identified with her crying and somehow knew it was a result of his anger and domination. Not being able to talk back to him, I used to write him notes expressing my feelings. He responded minimally. The writings didn't work to create a dialogue, but the purging helped me cope with my feelings.

When I turned 18, as with many young people, I was eager to leave home and go to college, anxious to leave the grip of my father's rigidity. In the fall of 1964 I went to Michigan State University in East Lansing. After graduating in June of 1968, I returned home briefly, then moved to Detroit in September of 1968 and married Jim McAndrews that December.

During the years from 1968 to 1975 the relationship with my parents was long distance. My husband and I lived in Detroit and saw them only three or four times a year. Wanting to "make it on my own," and still being somewhat rebellious, I needed this time of being separate and removed. It was a time of experimenting with life-styles and learning about the world. My husband and I were both social workers in Detroit, and I was learning about a world I had not known before. The realities of poverty, crime, and social injustice became readily apparent.

While I was still facing these realities and going through the first few years of married life, my father was getting ready to retire. I could see that he needed to do so as soon as he could. Even though he was very good at what he did, the stress of being a disciplinarian for 400-plus high school students was taking its toll.

I remember many times at dinner my mother taking the phone off the hook so we would not be bothered. Someone was frequently calling with a problem; perhaps a teacher being sick and needing a substitute, or a student's parent realizing that his or her child was having problems. My father was a dedicated school administrator, but the stress of the job began to affect his health. My mother remembers many times when he would go to work sick and feverish. He should have stayed home, but his workaholic self believed no one could do the job as well as he could.

Finally he retired. In the summer of 1970 my parents moved to Arcadia in northwestern Michigan. My father had always been a strong man and inclined to hard physical work, which he enjoyed almost as much as his administrative duties. He took on the job of maintenance man and caretaker for Camp Arcadia, a Lutheran summer camp on the shores of Lake Michigan. He seemed to enjoy the work, but it was always hard to tell whether he was really enjoying anything. He was so compulsive about work that everything he did could turn into a serious task to be tackled and accomplished to its most efficient degree.

I think he was happy to be away from school responsibilities and to be back closer to where he had grown up. Being around people of his own religious tradition must have comforted him, and the work was satisfying.

Looking back on those years after his retirement from school, I don't see evidence of a change in him. My mother, however, says she thinks the beginnings of Alzheimer's may have been evident as early as 1970, because he began to say he "just couldn't do the job anymore." The job may have been difficult for anyone and the stress high, but perhaps there was the beginning of the disease process. Had we kept a diary detailing my father's actions, we may now have had more clues as to its beginnings. However, pinpointing the disease's onset remains difficult, if not impossible. Just as the neurofibrillary tangles of the victim's brain become more and more dense and tangled, so does a discussion about the onset of Alzheimer's disease.

The caretaker work in Arcadia lasted a little over a year, and in October 1971 my mother and father moved permanently to the house we had always used as a summer retreat when living in Battle Creek. It was located in Leelanau County, where they were born, in the Little Finger of Michigan in the northwestern part of the state. Each had been born and reared there and they had met each other as children. My mother can't remember a time when she didn't know my father. The home was outside of Maple City, a small town 15 miles northwest of Traverse City. My parents expanded the cottage and made it a permanent home.

I was sad when the old hand pump was torn out of the kitchen and modern plumbing was put in. I was sad when they covered up the old pink insulation with drywall. The romanticism of my youth was now gone. My younger brother Paul and I used to lie on the old bunkbeds, staring at the old pink insulation, telling stories or reading comic books. A modern house now replaced the rustic dwelling my dad and his brothers had built. We had always called it "the little house." "We're going up to 'the little house' for the weekend," we would say. But, of course, my parents for their retirement didn't leave it as it was. They had it remodeled and in the fall of 1971 moved in. I think they enjoyed themselves during those early retirement years. They were active in church activities, had many friends, and enjoyed gardening and working around the remodeled and expanded house, which they had never been able to enjoy full-time before. Many times my father had been back at school when my mother and Paul and I were still "up north" in the summer. Most of my father's family was in the area, too. He enjoyed visiting and being with his sisters and brother and their families. My father had gone home again.

As much as I never thought it would be, "going home again" became appropriate for me as well in 1975. About a year earlier, my father had helped me acquire some property from my cousin. It was located only about a mile from where my parents lived. The wooded location is where my husband Jim and I still make our home. During this time we bought a house from Sleeping Bear Dunes National Lakeshore and moved it to the property for a fraction of the cost of a new house. Jim was busy with his job and other things, so I took on the major portion of the preliminary dealings. I remember well all the business transactions I had to go through to bid on the house and have it moved and the respect I gained in my father's eyes as a result of doing so. Whatever male chauvinism he had exhibited, which had been a great deal, was eroded, at least in my relationship with him, after those transactions.

In August of 1975 I moved to this house in Leelanau County. My husband joined me five months later.

I remember fondly those times when we were trying to get everything ready for moving in; also, the projects we would work on around the house and the way my parents were both helpful with many things that needed doing — my mom with all of her canned fruits and vegetables, homemade baked goods, and fine home-cooked meals and my dad with his knowledge of carpentry and general maintenance. When he saw what I was using as a desk to do my work of court transcribing, he rushed home to his workshop and the next day delivered to me a desk, however primitive, the perfect height, width, and depth for my work. I have a new and fancier desk now, but the old one remains in my office.

I remember also a time when he helped Jim wire the basement. Jim would get exasperated at his compulsiveness, but the job got done to my father's enjoyment. During those years he also enjoyed cutting wood and other outside chores — cutting brush, clearing the field, planting the garden, doing general maintenance. He loved carpentry work and could make many pieces of furniture from scratch. He enjoyed working with his hands, which were rough and strong. Even in the last days of his life his handshake seemed as strong as it ever had been.

He stayed active in the church as an elder until the late 1970's and was on the Board of Review for the township until January 1979, when he told the township supervisor to find a replacement, since he "couldn't do the job anymore."

That was only the beginning of a long list of things my father would no longer be able to do.

Chapter III - Confusion

After the move to the newly remodeled home in northern Michigan, my father worked for the summer of 1972 as an assistant on a nephew's well drilling team. After the summer was over, he had to quit because he said he "just couldn't do it anymore" and he "just couldn't take orders from those young guys anymore," even though just the year before he had been able to carry out the caretaking duties at the summer camp. Was it his many other health problems (gout, nervous anxiety, dizzy spells, Meniere's disease) that caused his inability, or was it the beginnings of memory loss that made him drop out of yet another activity?

In 1972 my parents joined the local chapter of the Retired Teachers Association. After my father had been in the organization for a while, the president asked him if he would take the treasurer's job. He had handled numbers with ease, having been a math teacher for many years. Reluctant to accept the job, he finally agreed when my mother lovingly offered her assistance. After holding the job for two years he phoned the president and said he "just couldn't do it anymore." Once again Mother said she would help, even do it all, but he refused. When she asked him why, he never answered. I believe he probably just didn't know how and was ashamed to admit it. I'm sure he was extremely puzzled, almost mystified, at what was happening to him.

So many behaviors of Alzheimer's patients are attributable to other problems that it is difficult, even in retrospect, to label some actions with any degree of certainty. My mother remembers a return trip from Cincinnati where my father's sister lived. "We stopped at your house in Detroit," she recalls. "I don't remember what year that was, but it was 10:00 o'clock at night, and I thought we'd never make it, because the traffic bothered your father so much. I couldn't believe it, because he never complained about that before. And that was way back. I don't know what year." We determined the event must have been somewhere around 1973.

In 1973 my father had a prostate operation, a routine procedure for a man of 63. The doctor had instructed him to measure his urine after the operation. Following instructions, he urinated in a can to measure the output. My mother discovered that he was still using the can occasionally a year or more after the operation, so she put the can away. I remember him being obsessive and compulsive about many things, but this behavior was carrying things a bit too far. The puzzle remains as to what caused such behavior.

The review of my father's medical records reveals a list of many drugs used up to 1978: Isordil, Quiniglute, Dyazide, Benemid, Nitrostat, Valium, Halotestin, Ferrofolic, Erythrocin, Antivert, Azulfadine, Librax. Could the ingestion of all these drugs have contributed to the Alzheimer's? I continue to search for an answer, but I have yet to find one.

In July 1978 Pa's youngest child, my brother Paul, got married. Jim and I drove with the folks in their car to Baltimore for the wedding. Pa anxiously helped with the driving. At the wedding itself and throughout the weekend he was his familiar polite self, gracious to our hosts, the Blums, my sister-in-law Joanne's parents. Even though my father was having a difficult time accepting the fact that Joanne and her family were Jewish, he did remarkably well, especially when one considers his normally compulsive and dogmatic personality. He had been depressed prior to Paul's wedding and had taken to lying on the couch a lot. His activities had dwindled to eating, sleeping, and a little working when cajoled. I was surprised at his energy and pleasant attitude at the wedding. I had always thought that pleasurable events that one looked forward to helped the mental attitude. Now I had proof of my hypothesis. It seemed that lack of meaningful activities and goals made depression and degeneration progress more rapidly.

I remember my father's hypochondria. He worried about what would happen to him and thought every little pain was some fatal disease. He worried about his intake of salt and didn't eat much of it. He worried about dying of a heart attack, as his father had before him. He worried so much about his health that in the months of September, October, and December of 1978 he was admitted to the hospital three times with chest pain. Had he not been depressed before, the diagnosis of possible angina would have made him so. The September diagnosis was "arteriosclerotic heart disease with angina," then modified in October to "chest wall pain and possible angina." By December the doctor labeled it "most likely cardiac neurosis." A cardiac catheterization was scheduled for January of 1979 to confirm the accuracy of the diagnosis.

The year 1979 was difficult for my father. He had the cardiac catheterization as planned and was diagnosed as having what most people normally think of as hardening of the arteries. The hospital record states: "The patient is a difficult historian. It is difficult to get an exact description of these (chest) pains." His memory was failing.

On Sunday, February 2, his old beagle Browser was buried in the pines down the driveway from his house. My husband Jim did the digging. I remember my father staying in the house, afraid to go outside in the cold for fear he'd "catch something."

Often he even stopped himself from going to church, certain that a coughing person behind him, ahead of him, or beside him would give him a cold. The fear was a good excuse not to go anywhere. It became a self-fulfilling prophecy.

Visits to doctors in 1979 increased, including a March visit to a heart specialist three hours away. The conclusion of the many consultations was that he had low-grade diverticulitis, but that his chest pain problems were "probably skeletal-muscular, not heart related," and that he had "marked cardiac neurosis."

Spring of that year was the last time he helped in the garden, and again he said he just "couldn't do it anymore."

Mother remembers 1975 to 1980 as difficult, too. "He didn't want any company," she says. "And people would listen to him and not to me. I'd say, `Come anyway,' but people wouldn't come." He had always been an authority figure, and people did what he said. Apparently the reason he didn't want visitors coming was his inability to talk or be in a conversation with someone and understand it. My mother, however, says: "He didn't want people to come, but when they came, he would visit with them and he seemed to be happy to have them. And he didn't want to go anyplace, but if we did go anywhere, then he enjoyed it."

I recall many times during those years when we would be playing cards at the kitchen table and he would go in the bedroom and say he was sick and couldn't play. I think now he really left because he was simply forgetting how to play.

In October of 1979 a cousin got married in Muskegon, about a three-hour trip away, and he once again had difficulty driving in a strange city's traffic at night. Mother drove home at his request.

In November that year my parents went to California to stay for the winter with my older brother Jon, his wife Esther, and their three daughters. When my parents had said they would go to his house for the winter, Jon was surprised. My father had never stayed at one person's house, to visit, for more than three or four days. Then he would get up one morning at 4:00 a.m. and say it was time to go, that he had to get an early start.

My brother was finishing a large house he had started building in the mountains south of San Francisco. Jon was installing oak plank flooring in the family room and kitchen and encouraged Father to help him. He took the hammer in one hand, a nail in the other, looked at them, shook his head, and set them down. He couldn't put together what he was supposed to do. In my brother's words, "He seemed to know what to do, but could only sustain attention to it briefly. And because of that he got very frustrated."

During the time there he slept a lot. The doctor had prescribed Valium for him, and he would go to bed as early as 8:00 p.m. and sleep all night. Mother encouraged him to go for walks with her, but he only did it for one week and then quit. Two things he never seemed to tire of were eating out and going to church. He didn't seem to think of exposure to colds in California as a problem when attending church, perhaps due to the warmer weather, or perhaps he had just forgotten that particular phobia. Drives and social events he enjoyed, as long as he was not under pressure to remember names. He also liked the warmer climate in California. He played cards every night. He could still add and seemed to know what he was doing. He learned to run the microwave, but the intercom remained a mystery.

Jon knew our father was worrying about dying and perhaps knew his time was coming because he talked incessantly about his heart problems and his funeral. He mentioned to Jon what hymns were to be sung: "In the Garden" and "Rock of Ages." Later everyone was surprised to learn that Alzheimer's was what finally claimed him instead of the heart problems, the supposed presence of which had troubled him so deeply.

This trip was my father's first to California since Jon had moved there in 1976. He often had a hard time visiting his children in their homes. The control he so dearly cherished was diminished, if not totally usurped, when he was not in his own domain.

But, as Jon phrased it, our father, before dying, needed to come to grips with my brother's change in religious beliefs before he died. Jon had been ordained a Lutheran minister in 1960, then obtained a doctorate in religious studies at the University of Pennsylvania some years later in 1975. Jon's beliefs, at least in my father's conservative eyes, appeared to take a turn for the worse. As Jon saw it, at this time of his life our father was trying to piece together and understand his children before he left the world.

After he died, I asked Jon whether he thought the Alzheimer's or mental deterioration my father experienced somehow affected his ability to come to grips with the fact that his children did not hold identical religious beliefs. Jon had an interesting comment: "I think the same willpower that would have helped him sort out some of the conflicting elements in his own family might have helped him deal more effectively with the condition that became Alzheimer's. That isn't to say he would have been able to stop it, but he might have been able to prolong his life, because, if you know what's happening to you, you can sometimes hold out longer." Jon felt the disease had a great effect on our father's determination, without his knowing the cause. Perhaps his willpower would have been more focused had he understood early on what was happening. But in the end Jon said he felt it didn't matter if the disease was called Alzheimer's or not. "I knew that the basic problem was a running, a final running, toward his own death, and I felt bad about that. Death is the problem, and Alzheimer's just draws the process out longer." Philosophically speaking, his comment may be appropriate, but the physical realities of the disease prolong death unbearably and can tax the tempers of even the most patient.

The doctor's note for May 6, 1980, after the return from California in April, says, "Had flu and dizziness, but generally had a good winter."

Chapter IV - More Confusion

By June of 1980 my father's weight had dropped from 180 pounds to 141. Given that he was now only five-foot-seven, some weight loss was to his benefit, but at 141 pounds he did not resemble his stout, muscular, robust self. He had always loved to eat, and losing weight had never been an easy task. He had lost a third of the 39 pounds by going on a lowfat, low-salt diet at the doctor's suggestion, but to everyone's puzzlement the weight continued to come off.

Seeing my father growing older and feebler, in February 1981 I decided to preserve some of his memories. I started a project to tape his remembrances of ancestors and family in a series of interviews. (Later, after he died the tapes were difficult to listen to, but eventually they became a comfort.) It is interesting, though sad, to listen to examples of his confusion, memory loss, and misuse of words. In the first tape (February 1981) the instances are few in number. I discussed many of the schools where he used to teach. He remembered all of them and recounted stories with little misuse of words or sentence structure. When discussing some of his cousins whom he knew very well, but didn't remember the names of, he said, "Isn't that funny? I can't think of their names."

Three months after that interview, he entered a local hospital for extreme pain in his lower abdomen. He couldn't answer questions about his eating behavior or appetite and was unable to relate his medical history accurately to the admitting physician. Instead, he related that he had had "a heart attack in the past."

Perhaps all of his hospitalizations or chest pain had led him to believe he really had had a heart attack. One time he and my mother came to hear me sing at one of my early music performances, during which I sang and others played 12th to 16th century music on period instruments. Many friends were present. Afterward he talked incessantly about his recent "heart attack." Mother was embarrassed. I was surprised and took him aside and said, "Pa, you never had a heart attack." He looked at me blankly and said nothing, as if the last few minutes had not transpired.

A one-month hospital stay resulted from the abdominal pain. He had diverticulitis (an inflammation of an area of the intestinal tract) and had to have part of his colon removed. The hospitalization must have been a nightmare to him, at least when he remembered what he was and wasn't doing. The insidious nature of Alzheimer's leaves its victim babbling incoherently for several minutes or hours one day, with no awareness of the effect these actions have on those around him. Then later the afflicted person wonders at the memory loss, frustrated and puzzled at newly discovered lapses.

Although his physical condition could have caused some of the mental problems prior to this surgery, Alzheimer's patients do not do well when they experience a change in environment. My father was no exception. While he was in the hospital the week before the operation, the nurses' notes continually refer to him as being "very confused" or "somewhat confused as to time and place." One night he poured his medications down the drain. The same night he was unable to control his bowels and was very upset and ashamed about it. He was very efficient about cleaning himself up, but said he felt "like a pest." When the nurse or aide attempted to reassure him, he didn't understand what she said.

Once prior to surgery when my mother was visiting him, he stated to the nurse that he had "just let her take a nap" and that after 48 years of marriage you're content just to "dwell in one another's company." How true that phrase would be later on for my mother, when, even though he was at times unaware of her presence, she still was content to "dwell in his company." Later she would vacillate between wanting him whatever way he was and wanting his suffering to be over.

A few nights before surgery, at 4:30 a.m., he was found at his bedside standing by the IV pole, upon which was hanging his tube for intravenous medication and feeding. He was very confused about the IV pole and requested that it be dismantled.

On Saturday, May 23, at 7:20 a.m. he had a colon resection, a procedure in which part of the colon is removed. He tolerated the preparatory procedures and the operation itself very well. The doctor remarked afterward that he had a very strong heart, despite the earlier problems. By 7:00 p.m. that evening, after awakening, he was becoming restless and was thrashing about. More medication was given for the next several hours, but it did not seem to calm him. By the early morning hours he still had no urine output, his blood pressure was fluctuating, and his pulse was elevated. By 4:00 a.m. he had already been given eight units of blood.

At 5:00 a.m. Sunday morning my phone rang. It was my brother Paul saying the hospital had called and had indicated a need to reoperate because Pa was bleeding internally and his blood pressure was continuing to fluctuate.

I dressed immediately, and within minutes my mother and brother drove up my driveway in her car. She let Paul drive and said, "We had better say a prayer," which she proceeded to do. She looked very frightened. Perhaps few people are ever ready for a death, but we were definitely not ready for it to happen that day. The operation was supposed to be routine, and we were not expecting anything serious.

We arrived at the hospital after an aggravating 40-minute ride in the morning darkness. The attendants were taking my father into the operating room. I looked at his pale face and told myself not to worry.

My mother and I stayed in the waiting room and meditated, as we sometimes did together, using the technique to attain inner peace and greater energy. The act of meditation served to calm us, and I believed it might have a positive effect on my father in the operating room, just as some people believe prayer can. Paul went to talk to the nurses to find out what he could about my father's condition.

In a couple hours the operation was over. The doctor said my father was stable and was going to be all right. At 9:30 Pa started to talk and move. Greatly relieved, we saw him briefly and then went home. Paul and Mother went to church. We came back at 7:00 p.m. The staff said he had become restless later that afternoon and asked for help to get up. He apparently had not realized he had had surgery. He was still restless when we arrived.

Although some nurses' notes of the next two to three weeks indicate he was "alert, well oriented, up and about," most of them tell about his extreme confusion and anxiety. The first few days he had constant supervision. But when his surgical wound healed well enough for him to be able to get up, he was constantly asking the nurses to help him. He got up at his bedside. He walked to the nurse's station. He rang his bell. He asked that they come in and cover him up. Or he asked for help but then could not tell them what he needed help with. Many nights he was up intermittently all night.

During some of my visits we went for walks in the hall. He needed exercise, and the walking gave us something to do together. We would go to the end of the hallway, then turn around and come back. Several times I asked if he would like to go outdoors, since the weather was warm and pleasant. He looked at me like a frightened child, then turned around and walked the other way; he emphasized, "No!" When I asked "Why?" he wouldn't answer. At the time I thought depression caused his reticence. Now I realize he was probably afraid he would get lost and not be able to find his way back.

On May 31, 1981, a Sunday, he spent a very restless night. He was tucked in several times, saying each time he needed his covers adjusted. His conversation made no sense. As one nurse put it, "His mouth can't say what his brain is telling him." He "got out of bed, sat down on the bed, laid down, covered himself up, threw the covers off, and got out the other side."

The next night his restlessness got worse. Monday evening we went to visit him, and my mother told him of my sister Darlene's surgery. She had had a hysterectomy that morning. Mother told him she was all right. He didn't mention anything about it, but remained agitated and disoriented. At 8:00 p.m. his pulse was fluctuating and at 9:30 p.m. the doctor was notified. Extra medication had to be given. Even with the extra medication, he was still rambling and roaming in the hallways all night. He laid down, then called for the nurse and said, "I need help getting covered up." When asked if he considered getting up every 30 to 60 seconds made sense, he said, "No, it doesn't. I won't do it again. I want to be a good person."

Then five minutes later he did it again. That night he had visual hallucinations. He asked the nurse, "Do you see that picture on the wall?" And none was there.

That night was his worst so far in the hospital. I wonder if the news of my sister's operation upset him more than usual. Since he could not verbalize his problem, we didn't know what was troubling him. Already the process of dementia was having an effect.

A psychologist was called in because of my father's failure to return to a normal behavior pattern. The psychologist's analysis, full of psychological jargon, was that the behavior could be categorized as a "brief reactive psychosis, with a possible organic or dementia component," meaning that his loss of contact with reality could be a reaction to his hospital stay, but that the mental deterioration might have a physical cause. The psychologist even mentioned the possibility of suicide because of the depression.

The difficulty of diagnosis here became apparent. My father had many doctors at his disposal, and none of them even suggested the possibility of Alzheimer's disease. In 1981 there was little awareness, even on the part of doctors, of the distinction between the different diseases associated with dementia.

The entire staff at the hospital was very competent, but one male nurse in particular gave a little extra. He talked at length with my father, helping him with reality orientation and informing us of everything that was happening. He also took extremely detailed notes. On Thursday, June 4, at 3:30 p.m. my father was at the nurse's station once again. The nurse took him to his room, and the following dialogue ensued, according to the nurse's notes:

Mr. D.: Help me, please.
Nurse: What do you need help with, Mr. Dechow?

Mr. D.: I need help getting into bed.

Nurse: I feel you can get into bed by yourself, Mr. Dechow.

Mr. D.: I suppose I can, but I want you to help me do it, please.

Nurse: No. I want you to do it yourself. You should become independent. Do you have something bothering you, Mr. Dechow? Something you would like to talk about now?

Mr. D.: Yes. I have something bothering me. I don't know enough to be able to do this.

Nurse: Mr. Dechow, what can you tell me about where you are and what you have had done lately?

Mr. D.: Well, I'm in the hospital in Northport. I don't know the proper title. I came here to die.

Nurse: You say you came here to die.

Mr. D.: That's right. I'm not afraid to die.

Nurse: I don't feel that you came here to die. You came here because you had diverticulitis. Then the doctor did surgery on your colon. You can see the incision here on your abdomen. Do you remember having diverticulitis?

Mr. D.: Yes, I do. You know, I don't feel I know enough to do anything anymore.

Nurse: You say you don't feel you know enough to do anything anymore?

Mr. D.: I was a teacher of mathematics and social sciences. Then I was a school principal.

Nurse: That must have required a great deal of education. Do you feel that you can feed yourself and go to the bathroom and get into bed without assistance?

Mr. D.: I guess I could do that.
Nurse: Good. It is 4:10 p.m. now. I'll be back at
4:30 p.m., no sooner, no later, and I want
you to either sit in the chair or lie here in bed
until I get back.
Mr. D.: Okay. I'll do that.

The note for 4:30 indicates that this tactic of the nurse seemed to work. After that episode he was oriented and did not go back and forth to the nurse's station for a while. We came in to visit him at 4:45 p.m. and he recognized us and talked freely. The nurse had used very direct statements about the date, the time, and the consequences of his actions. This type of reality orientation worked for sometimes long periods of time. Since the Alzheimer's patient must constantly look for something concrete in a now disoriented world, simple statements provide clarity in an otherwise muddled situation. I came to use this technique many months later with my father, when his condition had worsened.

However attentive this nurse or any of the other nurses were, they could not watch my father constantly. The hospital was not equipped for such care. The next several days my father did not improve mentally. One nurse wrote on Friday, "He appears very rigid and trembles at times when assisted to bed. He climbs in on his hands and knees and then buries his head in the pillow and forgets to relax his trunk into bed." His positioning was almost catatonic. The next day the nurse asked him if he wanted to go for a walk, to which he replied, "Yes. Let's get out of here." The nurse grasped his hand tightly and walked with him to the day room, but when they arrived he wanted to go back to his own room.

We visited him late that afternoon. He recognized us, but was frightened and wanted us to stay all night. We told him we couldn't do that. He repeated the request again and again. Perhaps he felt that his lucid moments were slipping away, and he didn't know how much longer he would know us. On this day the nurse suggested that, if his behavior continued as it had been, we might want to look for another facility better equipped to handle mental problems. We didn't know what to do, but said we would discuss it with the doctor.

During this hospital stay his weight was somewhere between 130 and 140 pounds. He looked very frail and much older than his 70 years. One doctor commented that he was "eating everything on his plate," but still was "not getting enough calories." The problem with weight loss is common with Alzheimer's patients. They never seem to get enough to eat.

The rest of his hospital stay was more of the same. At times he was incontinent without realizing it. One time he had his pants off, and his gown was in knots. He started drooling. I wiped the drool off for him whenever I saw it. He appeared disturbed and puzzled about my actions. Several times he dumped his Ensure, a high-calorie food supplement, in the wastebasket. One time he even asked the nurse to dump some of his meal for him.

On Tuesday, June 9, he was found urinating on the floor. When questioned whether he knew he did it, he replied, "I certainly wouldn't do a thing like that."

Two days later, on Thursday, he was taken to another hospital for a CAT scan of his brain, a detailed type of x-ray which can sometimes assist in a clinical examination. When it was explained to him why he was going, he said, "It sounds like a good idea to me." The impression later was "No definite abnormality," but there was a questionable small infarct, or area of tissue which was dying or dead. Nothing, however, offered an explanation for the extent of his confusion.

The following afternoon he grabbed a nurse's hand, held the hand up to his face, and tried to make the nurse slap him. The nurse said, "I won't allow you to make me hurt you." The same staff person reported that he was "fragile or about at the breaking point and seemed about to cry."

During the previous few days we had talked to the doctor about my dad's state of mind. The doctor thought that the best thing to do would be to get him home and see if familiar surroundings would help him come back to reality. He was to be released on Saturday, June 13. His wound from the colon operation had sufficiently healed so that a visiting nurse could tend to it. The plan sounded appropriate.

On Friday, the day before his release, we came to see him. He jumped up and started to leave the room. The nurse told him to come back, to which he replied, "I will," but just kept walking away. When he finally did come back, he rambled on about dying in the hospital and said, "It's happened to others like this."

We reassured him that he was getting better and was going to live. My mother said, "You're not like the others." He said, "I'll fix it," jumped up, and flipped over his water stand, then laid down on the bed as if nothing had happened. After his tray was cleaned up, he insisted that Mother and I and the nurse sit where he told us, then expressed happiness about going home the following day.

That night he told the nurse he had talked to the doctor and to my mother about going home and wondered how it would "work out." His conversation was intelligible for a change, and he showed some understanding of what was happening.

Throughout his hospital stay, stability came from visits with family members. Even though he may have acted inappropriately on some visits, he recognized who we were and appeared pleased we were there. Going home held out hope that his mental faculties would return.

My mother and I came on Saturday morning to pick him up. He still looked very frail, but expressed pleasure at the thought of going home. On the way home we stopped for ice cream. He had to be told constantly what we were doing. When we got in the ice cream parlor, luckily there weren't many people around. He tried to walk out just as we got inside, but finally understood that we were getting ice cream. He took some money out of his wallet, what appeared to be all the money in his wallet, and handed it to me, saying, "Here. Use this." His awareness of the cost of ice cream was nil. I appreciated his need to pay his own way and treat us to ice cream, but his sense of how much things cost was not intact.

I obtained the ice cream from the proprietor and handed my father the cone. He walked around the store eating the ice cream like a little child who had never seen the stuff before. He ate voraciously and would have eaten a bigger helping, but he could not sit still. Mother and I tried to sit down and have him do the same, but he would have none of it. Walking was necessary right then; so he got up and ate the ice cream on foot. I was thankful that he knew who we were and that he was already acting better after leaving the hospital. He seemed anxious to get home and was delighted by the treat. The rest of the drive home consisted of reassuring him that we were going home and that his health would improve.

The doctor had been right. Getting my father home was the best thing we could have done for him. He was still recuperating from a serious operation. Recuperation took time, but he did improve. With Mother's great care and the visiting nurse's attention to his wound, his mind returned to a state approaching normal, although he still exhibited signs of depression and complained that he couldn't remember things. We would say, "You'll remember soon. You've been through a serious operation, and it takes time to recover."

He was still frightened of people. The first time the visiting nurse came, two days after his discharge from the hospital, he wouldn't let her come within five feet. The following day he let her change his dressing. With shoes and clothes on, he weighed 130 pounds. He was still preoccupied with his health and depression and had a very short attention span. From one day to the next he could not remember the nurse's name. He asked her several times what her name was and still was not sure of it. However, he was more able to follow conversations and appeared more alert.

On Friday, June 25, I took him to a psychiatrist on the recommendation of the visiting nurse and the doctor. He didn't understand what we were doing, but I told him that this doctor would perhaps be able to help him. In the mental status exam his answers were not appropriate. When asked to count backward from 100, he first said "73 or 37," then responded "93, 96, 97, 77, 70, 73." When asked about a few proverbs, specifically what "A stitch in time saves nine" meant, he replied, "Make correction before completely lost; we have done the job right." He was trying, but could not get the words right. It's as if he knew what he wanted to say, but could not formulate it into grammatically correct sentences.

When asked who the last five presidents were, he became upset and said, "Jimmy Carter and the guy who was shot," then said "Reagan" and a few names that made no sense at all. When asked to name some big cities, he replied, "New York. New York. San Francisco. Chicago. New York I forgot to name." The doctor's note says, "Recent and remote memory gone." His impression was "organic brain syndrome," a term so broad he may as well have said "senility." It didn't help us deal with what was to come, and we still didn't know what was wrong with him.

A few weeks later the visiting nurse noted that he was gaining in short and long term memory abilities and that, "Increased social stimulation has improved his speech patterns and social ability." Mother was helping him re-learn personal hygiene habits and encouraging him to participate in household activities. One thing he did a lot of was washing dishes. Mother kept saying she was going to buy a dishwasher. He didn't want to spend the money; so with guidance he continued to help with dishes.

The visiting nurse saw my father at least weekly until her discharge of him on August 12, 1981. By that time his weight had increased to 148 pounds, his appetite was very good, and he seemed to be returning to normal. He was still lying on the couch a lot, but was participating in some social activities. In late July of 1981 our family had a large reunion with many family members from as far away as Washington, and my father appeared to enjoy himself. He talked animatedly with relatives and told stories from the past.

On July 23 I taped a family get-together. We were at my parents' house. Everyone was sitting around the table after eating dinner. He again complained of not being able to remember things, but was at ease with many family members present. He often changed the subject when other people were talking, making me exasperated. Even in his illness he was manipulative. The hard part was discerning which times he was being manipulative and which times he was innocently forgetting something. In recounting the ordeal of the operation, which he did over and over again ad nauseam, he said, "You know who was the closest? My son Paul." When reminded of how often Mother came to see him, often almost every other day, he looked blank. Paul had been attentive, but living in Ann Arbor at the time, he was not there as often as Mother had been. The words of a memory impaired person can cut to the quick, and the perpetrator has no inkling of the effect his outbursts have on those he loves the most.

Mother was loyal despite the unintended barbs. In another recording taken by a friend in February 1982 Mother filled in the blanks with words he could not think of. As if in a game, he would pass the ball to her by saying, "Vi, you gotta help me," and she would comply lovingly. For some things she could be his memory.

The following are excerpts of a recording I took in January 1982. He was telling me about his grandfather who had his arm shot and rendered useless in the Civil War.

John D.: He didn't do anything for a long time, because he couldn't write anything with that right arm. And — what do you call men who took care of other men? I can't think what they're called. You know.

Lynn: You mean doctors?

John D.: I'm not thinking of doctors. I'm thinking about the other way. Those who were real good to them and preached to them and all that.

Lynn: Ministers?

John D.: Not ministers. Aren't they called something else, what they are today?

Lynn: I don't know. I don't know what you're talking about.

John D.: Well, when you do something for somebody else and they save your life and read to you and feed you?

Lynn: A nurse.

John D.: Jon signed up for one of them when he was a young man; our Jon.

Lynn: To be a minister, don't you mean?

John D.:   Not — it wasn't a minister. It was — you can call him an attendant, but that isn't what they called them. That's where the name began. What do you call a young man who went into the group of fighting men?

Lynn: Medic.

John D.:   Not a medic, but there's a combination.

Lynn: Oh.

John D.:   Where he prayed for them and he did things for them. What do you call them?

Lynn: Yeah. I think I know what you mean, but I can't think of the word either.

John D.:   What do you call them, Lynn? (Frustration in his voice)

Lynn: I can't think of it either. That's all right. It doesn't matter. So anyway somebody was taking care of him for a while before he came home?

John D.:   A man to serve him, to write his letters, helped him. And this man would send letters back to his home in Port Oneida.

Lynn: Oh, so he wasn't writing his own letters, then?

John D.:   No.

Lynn: Those letters were written by somebody else?

John D.:   Well, what's that somebody else called?

Lynn: I don't know.

John D.:   Yes, you do.

Lynn: I can't think of it.

John D.:   What are they called today when they go into the Army and they pray for people and they take care of them? I can't think of what they're called.

Lynn: I can't think of it either.

John D.: Men were hired to handle the wounded and the dying. And he stayed — he was there for several months.

Lynn: I remember reading some letters that were written from the war. You're saying those — he didn't write those? Somebody else wrote them?

John D.: Somebody — this person or one of these people wrote the letter back to his home. When he finally — when the war was over, or during the time that President Lincoln — what was the name of the place where he was shot?

Lynn: Ford Theater.

John D.: When Lincoln was at Ford Theater, Johann Heinrich Dago (early phonetic English spelling of the German "Dechow" name) was at the Spotsylvania Courthouse, and he was keeping guard there.

The word he had been desperately trying to think of was probably chaplain. Oddly enough, at the time I couldn't remember it either, so was of no help to him.

Later, when speaking of the parents of his mother Zena (nee Steiger), he misused words that he never would have in the past:

> Joseph Steiger had some way had got a *homeship* on that place through people giving it to him. They were related in some way to my own mother; those people that granted that piece of ground to Joseph Steiger.
>
> Grandmother Steiger died in 1918 in the wintertime. It was in the — if I remember correctly, and I don't remember correctly. Keep that in *vogue*, that I don't remember very *closely*, but it was in the wintertime, and my — and I think it was during the month of February when she died.

About his mother's death, this exchange took place:

John D.: Now, the next morning I was with my father
          feeding the chickens and so on, and we went by
          the *cluck*— coop, and three of — one, two, or
          three of those *clucks* got out and they *cloved* —
          they made the same noise as a rooster.
Lynn: Crowed?
John D.: They crowed like a rooster. My father grabbed
          one of them and picked it up. He chopped his
          head off. He was going to have him for dinner.

The consternation in his voice still lives in my memory.
He would say, "Confound it, Lynn. I can't remember
that," or "Goll darn it." Or, on the other hand, he would
say, "One particular case I shall *always* remember is the
choir I attended at the university." "Always" is illusory.

His short term memory appeared to improve in the
months following the operation. As time went on, we
noticed the problem less, because there was now a world
of difference from the man who had been in the hospital
in May. The lapses were still occurring, but were subtle
and infrequent.

In March 1982 my father drove to Traverse City with
my mother in the car. According to her he went over the
centerline on a busy street. Snow covered the road, and
the centerline was almost impossible to see. A policeman
stopped them and gave him a ticket.

In May he received a statement from the Secretary of
State's office saying that he would have to appear that
month and again in August for a driving test. I helped
him study the booklet put out by the State of Michigan,
"What Every Driver Must Know."

"Lynn, go over that part again," he pleaded. I thought
he was just trying to refresh his memory so he could pass

the test. I didn't know it then, but the whole book had become a puzzle to him. He feigned understanding and struggled with the basics of Michigan traffic law, desperately seeking to hold onto one of the last vestiges of his independence.

One day in July, toward the end of his time for hopeful study, we walked together on the gravel road in front of his house. It was a beautiful summer evening, the vista full of fresh wildflowers and the smell of greenery in the air. But he noticed none of this beauty. He had work to do.

I held the book in one hand and his hand in the other and quizzed him. "What does this sign mean?" I held up the book and showed him a diamond shaped yellow sign with two arrows in it, one pointing up and one down. He told me what he thought it meant. If he was wrong, I repeated it or corrected him. His right answers were very few. When he responded correctly, I gave him much praise, as he often had to me in a learning situation. "Is that enough of that one now?" I queried. Eyes downcast, feet shuffling, he replied, "You better do that one again, Lynn. I just can't remember very well anymore." I repeated the item and any others he desired until it was time to go inside.

I had no idea about the extent of his driving difficulties. I had recently witnessed him operating the controls, but many times when I was with him someone else might be driving. We are fortunate that his driving was stopped when it was. The horror stories of Alzheimer's victims having car accidents or losing their way in a morass of streets which now look like a maze are better left to the imagination. In August, when he went in for the driving test, the examiner told him that he could not drive anymore and his license was revoked. His depression continued.

Chapter V - Deterioration

In early September 1982 I interviewed my father again, asking him to recount stories about his aunts, uncles, and parents. He gave many "Yes's" and very short answers. He needed more prompting and did not volunteer as much as before. As part of one answer, he desperately tried to think of the word for the local nursing home. Finally, he settled on "the place where they have games and so on." Little did he know that in a year and a half he would be a resident. Aided by my mother, I asked him about his own mother's brothers and sisters and then his stepmother's brothers and sisters. His mother had died when he was only 10.

Lynn: How about your stepmother Dechow? Did she have any brothers and sisters?

John D.: What do you mean, "stepmother"?

Lynn: Well, after your mother died, then your — Anna Dechow's? Did she have any brothers and sisters?

John D.: Who? Anna?

Lynn: Yeah.

John D.: Well, I told you the brothers and sisters, dear.

Lynn: No. This is your mother Zena. I'm talking about your stepmother Anna.

Viola D.: Ed.

John D.: Well, I told you all the people.

Viola D.: Ed and Joe, and what was Mrs. Kilway's name?
Lynn: I'm talking about Anna Bufka.
John D.: Oh. I don't know very much about them. (He knew a lot about them)
Lynn: Joe and Ed and Mrs. Kilway, whatever her name was. Is she dead?
Viola D.: Yes. What was Mrs. Kilway's name? Lawrence's mother.
John D.: You'll just have to ask one of them, one of the Bufkas. I don't know.
Lynn: All right.
Viola D.: You know her name, Pa.
Lynn: That's all right. I —
John D.: I don't either know her name. I'd say it if I know it.
Lynn: Joe's still alive. Is Ed still alive?
Viola D.: It'll come to me.
John D.: Ed is — no. He's dead.
Viola D.: Carrie. Her name is Carrie.

For the moment my mother had won. She had remembered the name for him. She would help, sometimes lovingly, sometimes frustratedly, as if pleading with him to be able to remember. But he couldn't.

Even his memory for doing the dishes escaped him, and he had to ask Mother to help him. By asking her assistance rather than instruction, he watched and saw what to do and didn't have to admit that he didn't know how.

During 1982 his fear increased. He had often been fearful, but now his panic worsened and logical explanation had no effect. One time Mother was taking a walk in the woods by herself, which she did occasionally in late summer and early fall, looking for blackberries. She had told me earlier in the day that she had planned to go. Many times he would try to stop her by saying he was sick. Finally, after he "cried wolf" one too many times, she decided to go anyway. If he had had his way, she would never go anywhere. He would say, "Vi, I'm really sick," or do something that would show need for her to stay home.

About a half hour after she had been outside, he called me and said, "Lynn, Ma hasn't come home yet. Do you think I should call the Sheriff?"

"No," I replied. "She'll be home shortly. Don't worry about it."

Ten minutes later he called again and pleaded, "She's not home yet. What am I going to do?" He was near tears.

"No," I responded. "I'm sure she's fine and will be home soon."

Ten minutes elapsed, and the phone rang again. I knew who it was. I became firm with him and said, "I'm working. Please don't call me anymore. If she's not home in a half hour, I'll take a walk and look for her." As always, she returned home, and in their interaction he gave no indication that he had been worried.

Reports from others indicated that he had called other people when she was not at home. He may have called the sheriff half a dozen times that day. We know he talked to the oil man and had him deliver oil when the tank would only take less than 20 gallons. Mother had to pay a surcharge for the delivery, because it was less than the minimum order.

In late October or early November my brother Paul was visiting. He asked my father to show him the back of their property so that he could post "No Hunting" signs. Father lay on the couch and said he didn't want to go. After Paul's convincing, they drove on a gravel road to the two-track on the back of the property, then walked a few hundred yards to the property line. Agitated, Father wanted to leave as soon as he got there. "Put a sign on that tree," he directed, but it was as if he was telling Paul to place it indiscriminately so they could leave sooner. It occurred to Paul: *"Maybe he just doesn't know where he is back here."* For a city person disorientation in the woods would not be surprising, but my father had hunted and walked in that area for most of his life.

Paul remembers him saying that his "memory was shot." Paul mused that none of us took him literally. The statement was so simple that no one realized its significance. Not only was he saying he couldn't remember the name of a dish, he couldn't recall how to pick it up, dry it, or put it in the cupboard either. When he said, "I can't do that anymore," he meant, "I can't remember how to do it anymore." Perhaps had we shown him exactly what to do instead of trying to tell him repeatedly, the frustration for all of us may not have been so great.

One person who did show him exactly what to do was my sister Darlene's husband, John Sims. He would tell him exactly what to do or have the task laid out for him. He'd say, "Eat this piece of meat with this fork," or even feed him if necessary. Short, simple commands occasionally worked. In early December 1982 my parents went to Tampa, Florida, to stay with the Sims for the winter. When my father had suggested to Darlene in July that they come down, she was surprised. His desire to stay was out of character, for he had refused her earlier invitations except for short visits and family weddings.

In November I had the opportunity to go to Europe for six weeks as a companion for a friend and her children. One day in Paris I spotted an article in the science section of *The International Herald Tribune* about a disease called Alzheimer's. It was the first time I had heard of it. The behavior described sounded frighteningly familiar: "memory loss, learning and concentration disabilities, disorientation in time and space, inability to communicate,

poor coordination, and startling personality changes."
Immediately I mailed the article to my mother. *"Could this
be what plagued my father?"* I wondered. The author,
Nadine Brozan, talked of research being done on the disease, but gave no hope of any cure in the near future.

The interviewee spoke of the devastation that isolation
had on its victims. "Nobody comes to visit us anymore,
nobody calls, everybody ducks us. People are afraid." I
felt a chilling recognition as I read those words. Even
those few who still wanted to visit my folks stayed away
because my father told them to.

After my duties as companion were over, ending in
Paris, I traveled alone for a few weeks in southern France.
I flew back to New York and visited a friend for a few
days, then returned to Michigan.

Upon arrival at Detroit Metropolitan Airport, I eagerly
met Jim, who had driven from our home to meet me. This
was the first time in many years we had been separated for
more than a few weeks. Homecoming felt sweet. I
laughed and talked about the glories of travel and rode
down the escalator to find my suitcase. Abruptly, I noticed at the bottom a frail looking, white haired man, with
a one or two day's growth of white whiskers, talking animatedly to the security guard. I couldn't discern exactly
what he was saying, but he appeared frightened and
seemed to be asking the guard, "What do we do now?"
and "Where should I go?" I got close enough to say
"Hello." My father greeted me, then went right on talking to the guard, asking for help. I took his arm and said
we would be leaving soon.

The guard looked at me, gave a knowing look, and
went about his business. I appreciated that he wasn't
rude to my father, as some would be in that situation. An
airport baggage pickup center does not help the reality
orientation of a dementia victim. The sights and sounds

of hundreds of people milling about, a loudspeaker overhead, and lights glaring can be stressful to anyone.

Part of my father's personality hadn't changed. He often introduced himself, forthrightly asked questions of those who seemed to know, and told complete strangers his life story, whether they wanted to know it or not. He discovered much information that way. One time he met a man on a bus, whose family later hosted me for a week in England in elaborate style solely on the strength of my father's talkative nature.

Now, however, the gregariousness was all that seemed to remain. The inappropriateness of the questions and the fear exhibited on my father's face left me, on the one hand, nervously laughing to keep from crying and, on the other, directing him as one would a child, reluctant to play the parent role just yet.

From the airport we went to Paul's and Joanne's apartment in Ann Arbor. Jim and I returned home to northern Michigan the following day. My parents flew with Paul and Joanne to Tampa, where they were going to spend the winter with Darlene and John Sims. Paul says he noticed that Father had an odor about him, as if he hadn't had a bath in a while. Paul talked to him about it, but Father didn't understand and became frustrated because of Paul's scolding.

Due to a misunderstanding, the four of them waited at the Tampa airport for over an hour for someone to pick them up. My father kept wandering around, saying the same thing over and over, counting the bags repeatedly to make sure they were all there. Paul dutifully followed him when he started walking for fear he would not find his way back.

Upon arrival at John's and Darlene's house, my father needed constant reassurance and wanted someone nearby to help him sort out the confusion his new surroundings were fast becoming. Their house was a large one-story brick building that included, attached to the garage, a separate small apartment, with bedroom and bath, where my folks stayed. The main house was large with many rooms. Father had been there many times before, but now needed orientation as if to new surroundings. My sister had five children, all of whom were adults by this time. Two daughters were still living at home: Laree, the youngest, and Vicki, the middle child. Their boyfriends were at the house often, in addition to Cristi, the next youngest, and her husband Mark. My father loved his grandchildren. But since there were so many, a family joke had been made of the fact that, if he couldn't remember someone's name, he would say, "Vicki, Cristi, Laree, or whatever your name is." Now the mixup with names was no longer a joke. He might laugh nervously when a name didn't come out right, but fear dominated his emotions.

John and Darlene had lived in Florida for several years. Before they settled there they had moved many times. John had been an officer in the Air Force, and every child had been born in a different state. Now Darlene was a school librarian and John was attending school to become certified as a school counselor. Soon all the children would be gone from home. They looked forward to having their parents stay for a while in the winter, as Michigan was a long distance and visits to it were infrequent. They weren't prepared, however, for the events of the coming few months.

If my father was left alone for even a few moments, he wandered around as if he wasn't sure where a door was or where he should be going. Occasionally he saw one of the granddaughters or their boyfriends sitting in a room and said to John, "Who is that person in there? Who is that?" Later, he didn't even recognize my sister Darlene.

In her words, one of the worst aspects of Alzheimer's disease comes when the victim or loved one "looks at you blankly and doesn't really know you."

"Our father who art in heaven. Hallowed be thy name...." The words intoned a solemn ritual. John was driving and Father rode in the passenger's seat. Mom and Darlene sat in back. No matter where they went in the car or how short the distance, Dad would pray incessantly because of the great fear he had now acquired of riding in a car. After a while the recitation became routine.

Shortly before Christmas John and Darlene took my parents to one of the local decorated homes open for public exhibition. Outside in the yard were holly boughs and greenery and mistletoe; inside were gifts wrapped in reds and greens and glittery paper, inviting one to enjoy the Yuletide season. Darlene took my father by the arm and said, "It's all right, Daddy. It's all right. You're with me." He was afraid. Each time she took a step she would explain where they were and what they were doing. For a few minutes he would appear calmed. Then the fear would return until the reassurance was repeated. As John put it, his only enjoyment came from "being close to somebody who was reassuring him."

During the visit to the Christmas house he wandered away from Darlene. He was still in the yard of the house, but acted as if he couldn't find his way back to the sidewalk in front. Darlene retrieved him and she began the reassurance again, as if for the first time.

Back at their house he wandered also — mostly indoors. A few times they found him outside in the yard. Luckily, with constant vigilance, he didn't venture beyond their property.

To dissipate some of his energy, my mother would take my father for walks every day. If left to go alone, he would get lost. One time he said insistently, "Vi, let's go down this street" — which was the wrong way to go. She said, "No," but he almost insisted. Afraid of becoming lost and being unable to persuade him to return, she had to stop the daily walks. One day they were passing a house when he looked at it and said, "We better move down here." His former self wouldn't have considered that thought.

In my father's case a very positive aspect of the disease came in the loss of some inhibitions. He had hardly ever gone swimming with us when we went as a family except perhaps in his younger days. Now, surprisingly, he jumped in the pool and frolicked as if he were a child discovering the joys of playing in the water for the first time. When he wasn't in the water, he sat in a lawn chair by the pool with his old cap on playing with my sister's two little dogs and calling them "Doggins."

He had always enjoyed playing cards. Over the winter, from December to March, his ability to play went from bad to worse. At first, confused, he missed things and couldn't remember all the rules. Then later he said he wanted to play, but had to be prompted for every move, such as, "Pick up your cards, put them in order by suit, play that one now." Finally, he couldn't even shuffle the cards. A month or so later he put the cards in his hand, some facing him, some facing away, not aware of the aberration. He looked around and didn't know when to play. One time he poured his glass of water into a plate, then nonchalantly placed his cards in the water.

In card playing, as in other activities, he wanted desperately to do it right. He aimed to please. In household activities he wanted to do his share. He tried to set the table. But with the attention span of a two-year-old, requests had to be repeated three times, and even then it was doubtful that he could comply. Even simple commands like my mother's "Get the plate out of the cupboard" were not understood.

When he did get the utensils as far as the table, at first he placed the napkins properly to the left of the plate underneath the fork. Later, he spread them out flat anywhere on the table. After a while, no one corrected this behavior. He was being useful, or trying to. Often it took more energy to help him do things than it did to perform the task. A few times John handed him the dish towel and a dish and told him to dry it. He stood there with the dish in one hand, the towel in the other, but no motion served to connect the two items. To him they were unrelated.

The act of sweeping with a broom around the pool remained connected for Pa. He had always loved to work outdoors. John showed him how to take the garbage out to the road, which he continued to do as late as January. But this proved to be a mistake, as he then knew how to exit the house and might wander off.

Money in his hands became a problem. He gave money to John for no reason. Usually my father had been a generous man, but now he acted as if he were playing Monopoly and there was no tomorrow. John returned the money to Mom, but she, ever hopeful, gave it again to Dad. The cycle repeated itself. John kept it until finally my father had given him all his money. Finally, Mom agreed not to entrust it to him anymore.

Earlier that year he had been a little too generous, but Mom couldn't stop him when he sold a few large items without telling other family members who might have been interested. As if he were no longer aware of the value of things, he sold his big John Deere tractor, complete with snowblower, for less than it was worth. He gave the rototiller and steel boat to Jim and me. He sold two acres of land for a nominal sum. If he reflected in his clear moments about his life, perhaps he knew his time was short. But the decisions on big items were too impulsive. He consulted Mom on the land — her name was on the deed — but with the other items he acted as if they were his alone. The situation could have been worse. She was able to keep the checkbook intact without his writing checks for large sums of money.

The many problems he was having were not for lack of trying to do otherwise. In December he made lists for himself to help him remember. He wrote down his address and phone number. He wrote down all the colleges he had gone to, thinking that if he could repeat them enough times, maybe he would remember them. He listed all the places he had worked. He made lists and carried them with him. A week or two after making the lists he looked at them and didn't know what they were. After he died my mother found more lists in his desk — names of his medications, names of places he had lived, dates of important events. I wondered at his verbal lists — he prayed every night and listed all his children and grandchildren whom he wanted to be blessed. That ritual had gone on for a long while. Now the praying served a functional purpose as well as a spiritual one. He had always loved to sing. In Florida he sat by John in church every Sunday and sang old familiar hymns.

He had always loved going to church and enjoyed fellowship with others. He met new people, sometimes thought he knew them from before. Still, he preferred to stay close to those he knew well.

On New Year's Eve there was a party at a cousin's house near Tampa. Dad had a very good time. There was a lot of good food, a big fire, friendly people. Darlene said he seemed almost like his old self. He laughed and joked and told stories that made sense. Perhaps the Auld Lang Syne atmosphere made his life easier momentarily. Maybe he was just having a good day.

But in the regular run of things, many of the basic components of living from one day to the next — eating, sleeping, bathing, dressing, going to the bathroom — were becoming monumental tasks. My mother would lay his clothes out for him, or else he might don four pairs of socks and two flannel shirts in 80-degree weather. He needed the bath water run for him so he wouldn't scald himself. The water temperature left no mark on his sense of touch, it seemed, even though it might leave a burn on his skin. Mom worried about fire in their bedroom, because he would unnecessarily turn the heater up. The temperature might be 88 degrees, and he would act as if nothing had changed. Near the first of the year John and Darlene put an intercom speaker in my parents' bedroom and left it on 24 hours a day so they could hear what transpired, especially in case she was asleep or not in the room.

In February my mother fell when getting out of the car and couldn't get up by herself. My father tried to take her hand and said, "Get up." She recalled later, "Ordinarily he wouldn't do a thing like that. He didn't understand, and he wasn't concerned at all anymore about what happened to me."

Thinking that she would be all right, she didn't go to the doctor for a few weeks. Later it was discovered she had a broken hip. Yet she did not have an operation until returning to Michigan.

Because she could not maneuver very well by herself and my father did not understand what had happened, she moved into the main part of the Tampa house; Dad remained in the outside room. He tried to get to her and coax her to walk or do things with him, none of which she was able to do. He could not understand the change in his best companion. She loved him, but she had had enough of his mental problems and needed to concentrate on herself for a change. With difficulty, Darlene and John kept him in his own section of the house.

Dad had had some trouble sleeping before, but now his disorientation to time increased. Many nights John found him outside after he was supposed to have gone to bed. My father thought it was daytime. John said, "Look at the stars, Dad. It's nighttime." Occasionally, the medication he was taking, Sinequan, helped him sleep all night, but he may not have been taking it every night. Pills were a problem with him. Mom had been administering them to him, then later John and Darlene did so. But after Mom hurt her hip, John and Darlene found them hidden under the mattress, on the window ledge, or behind clothes.

My mother thought perhaps one reason for my father's nocturnal waking was hunger, since he would usually eat dinner at 5:00 p.m. and go to bed by 8:00 p.m. John and Darlene started giving him his medication along with something to eat, especially his favorite ice cream and cookies, before they retired at 11:00 p.m. Perhaps he would sleep three or four hours instead of only a half hour, as he had done before. Many nights John was up with him six or eight times in one night. Once John found him sweeping near the pool at 3:00 a.m. He did his chores as if there was nothing unusual about the time he had chosen to accomplish them. He didn't even appear tired. He seemed to have an inexhaustible supply of nervous energy, while those who cared for him were running on low, close to empty. Mom had appeared tired when they had first arrived. Now John and Darlene were becoming exhausted as well.

Darlene described her feelings: "I thought I was going crazy. I was so stressed by the whole thing that one night I came home from choir practice and I couldn't remember how to turn my lights off in the car. John had to do it for me." Sometimes in the morning when Darlene was leaving for work, my father would come out the door and chase after her, getting as far as the driveway, and then would be unable to relate what he had wanted. She had to lead him back into the house before she could leave again.

Realism and acceptance were John's way of dealing with the stress and emotional tension of life with a dementia victim. As he put it, there was more effort involved in telling someone, "Now, don't eat your meat with your fingers," or "You remember, use your spoon for the soup," than there was in cutting the meat, holding the utensils, and feeding the person if necessary. Acceptance was perhaps more difficult for my mother and Darlene than for John, who was not directly related. He could be more objective here, even though he had a mother in a nursing home with the same sort of problems. Instead of asking, "What would you like to eat?" he would say, "Here's some meat. Eat it," or he would hold the fork for him.

As time went on, John spent more and more time with my father — feeding him, dressing him, leading him from place to place. His whiskers were allowed to grow so he wouldn't have to be shaved every day. John and Darlene bought him pants with a stretch waistband, because he couldn't remember how to unzip and unbuckle his pants when going to the bathroom. He went when you took him, but did not go of his own accord.

On March 21, 1983, John and Darlene, hoping for some illumination about our father's problems, took him to a neurologist in Tampa for an exam. In one test the doctor said, "I'm going to say three things, and I want you to repeat them back to me when I count to three." They were simple things like, "Fifty, a hat, a house. One, two, three. Repeat those back to me." My father replied, "Would you like to see my operation scar?" During the 20-minute exam many tests were given. Further evaluation was recommended to rule out "a metabolic problem and/or intracranial lesion." But the doctor stated his impression thus: "The patient's history is most compatible with a senile dementia." Once again, those two words were used, signifying nothing except that there was no hope.

By the time my father returned to Michigan on March 29 he barely knew anything of what was going on. John says if he had remained perhaps a few days longer, he may have had to return to Michigan by ambulance or he might have ended up in a nursing home in Tampa.

Except for his mindless, incessant talking to his seat companion, who looked as if he would rather be reading, the plane trip to Ann Arbor was relatively quiet. At both ends my parents were assisted by an escort and a wheelchair, since Mother could only walk with a walker, and then very slowly. She was to have an appointment to schedule a hip operation on Tuesday, March 29, at the University of Michigan Hospital, where my sister-in-law Joanne was a physician.

Darlene and John saw them off at the airport. Darlene looked at our father and saw that now familiar blank stare. She said goodbye. She's sure he didn't know who she was.

Chapter VI - Crisis

My folks arrived at the Detroit airport on Tuesday, March 29. My husband Jim was on hand to meet them. Mom was in a wheelchair and appeared very tired. My father looked distinguished with his now all white hair and beard. Jim met them in the lobby as they came from the plane. He was sure Dad recognized him. Generally aware of the surroundings, Dad was glad to be on his way home.

My father's confusion became apparent, however, when the time came to leave the airport and go to the car. He acted as if he understood little of what was happening. Jim explained that they were going to Paul and Joanne's apartment for a few hours to rest, and then were going to drive home to Maple City. The time was early afternoon, and Joanne was still at work. Paul was out of town, his absence possibly adding to Dad's confusion. There was time before Mom's appointment at University of Michigan Hospital for her hip; so Jim got them settled in for a nap. Mom asked Jim to run an errand for her. With both of them resting in separate rooms, Jim left.

Jim was gone less than an hour. As he pulled into the driveway of the complex, Jim saw my father talking animatedly with a man who appeared to be manager of the apartments. The manager had found him wandering from building to building. The apartment complex, located near a river, is large, with buildings, to a newcomer, all looking the same. Until one is used to the surroundings, going into the wrong building is easy. Dad was unable to tell the man how he got there, where he was going, or where he should be.

When Jim found them, my father did not seem excited or nervous about being lost. He simply could not remember where to go. The man left, reassured that Jim could lead Dad back home. Jim said, "We're at Paul and Joanne's place." He had to remind him who Paul was and that Mom was back at their apartment. Dad gave no resistance. As Jim labeled his demeanor, he was "benignly confused." When they returned to the apartment, Mom was happy he was safe. But she scolded him for leaving the apartment and not waking her up, since she had told him to if he awoke before she did.

Joanne took Mom to her appointment. Jim stayed with Dad. By late afternoon Dad's anxiety level had increased. He needed constant reassurance as to where he was and why. They had dinner with Joanne, and afterward, around 6:00 p.m., started the five-hour trip north. Jim had to be back on Wednesday for an appointment, or they might have waited until the next day to leave.

The first two-and-a-half hours of the trip were calm enough. Daylight was not gone, and tiredness had not as yet taken its toll on Dad. Mom sat in the back seat, Jim drove, and Dad also sat in the front. The second half of the trip, north of Clare, was "the longest trip" Jim "had ever taken." My father began to get confused and bewildered. He thought he could see landmarks at every crossroad. At every one he would advise, "Turn here. This is the way." When the car continued on a straight path, he'd say, "Why don't you turn here?" Jim explained many, many times to him that the suggestions were not correct and the trip would just take longer. Logical explanation made no dent in his insistence.

Jim told Dad, "I'd appreciate it if you would just let me drive." When Jim did not comply with the request to turn, Dad started to whimper and cry. Jim finally said, "Stop that. I don't want to hear the questions anymore." Mom said, "Now, John, just shut up." Dad stopped for a few minutes, then started again. He would not do it at imaginary paths or two-tracks; just crossroads. The words were first requests, then commands; then, when no response was forthcoming, anguished pleas. After 25 repeats, and no answer Jim could give would satisfy him, Jim said, "Dad, you don't seem to want to take my reassurances, and I've tried to tell you we are this far from home. Believe me, I know how to get there, and I'm trying to get there as quickly as I can. But it is going to take some time, and I just wish you'd be quiet for a while." This statement worked for a crossroad or two.

Then, as Jim put it, "It became obvious that he wasn't motivated by trying to give anyone a hard time. He was moving into a state of panic in which he was quite certain that this idiot driving the car was either deliberately trying to take him someplace or was just foolish enough not to take the right road. He understood the concept of home. I'm not sure he understood that to get home you had to do what we were doing."

About a half hour before arriving at my parents' home, Jim started reminding my father that he would be home soon and that they were going to his house. Jim pointed out various landmarks along the way. Dad didn't seem to recognize anything, including our house, which they passed about a mile before finally getting to their own home at about 11:00 p.m. As they were pulling into the long driveway to the house, Jim said, "This is your house." Dad said, "It is?" and then, "No, it's not." He got out of the car, looked around, and said, "Where are the people who live here? When are they coming back?" Jim and Mom both replied, "This is your house. We can go in and go to bed."

All three were exhausted, especially my mother, who just wanted to sleep. Jim helped her inside, then saw to Dad, who had by then seen all the family pictures on the piano. Jim reminded him that these were his children and grandchildren. He entertained the possibility briefly, then lapsed back into, "Where are the people who live here?" He was genuinely concerned that these people would return and he would be in big trouble. He commented about the police coming to get him.

Mom retired to the small bedroom off the kitchen to get ready for bed. She wanted no more of Dad's insanity. She was exhausted herself and needed sleep badly. Jim took Dad into Mom and Dad's former joint bedroom, which was at the end of the hall from the living room. Since getting him into his pajamas seemed an impossibility, Jim encouraged him to lie down. He refused. He was in a home that wasn't his and the people could return at any time. He wasn't necessarily trying to get to Mom, just to get out of the bedroom. Jim said firmly, "You can't go out. It's time to go to bed." Dad became frightened and infuriated. He called Jim a name and took a swing at him with his fist. He missed, but was clearly trying to hit him. Jim blocked the blow with his own arm, pinned Pa's arm behind him and threw him on the bed. Jim thought at the time, *"This guy is strong and could be a handful."* What he said was, "Don't you take another swing at me."

Mom had heard their voices and tried to help Jim again in getting Dad to calm down. Finally, both Mom and Jim, exhausted, sat at the kitchen table for a few minutes and talked about something totally unrelated to what was transpiring with Dad. Dad became more docile after Jim's forcefulness. He came into the room two or three times, mumbling under his breath. They ignored him. In Jim's words, "By that time he could have said anything, given a PhD dissertation, been the most logical person you ever met, and we wouldn't have talked to him."

Jim laid down on the couch for a while, then fell asleep. Mom did the same in her bedroom. Jim thought certain he would hear Dad if he did anything strange. Once Dad came out in the middle of the night. When Jim ignored him, he returned to the bedroom.

At 6:00 o'clock Wednesday morning our dogs suddenly started barking, indicating a possible visitor at the door. I went downstairs to the door and saw someone standing outside. It was my father, looking thoroughly distraught. He had his clothes on over his pajamas, with moccasins on his feet. His hair was uncombed, and he had a strange stare in his eye, making him look every bit a wild man. Little did I know how much wilder he would seem after the events of the next few weeks.

He muttered something about needing the sheriff and that his house wasn't right. He was very confused, and I could see that keeping him in the house was going to be difficult. I had talked to Jim the night before. He had been tired and did not want to elaborate on the details of the trip until he saw me, although he sounded as if he had been through an ordeal.

In short order I discovered what sort of problem Jim had faced on the trip. I hadn't seen my father since I had left for Europe last November, when he, Jim, and my mother had seen me off at the airport.

Now he seemed much more distant — frightened, vulnerable, like a child who had just learned to be afraid of a thunderstorm, or like a wild animal that was running for its life. He had walked from his house, which he no longer recognized, to mine. How he got there without

getting lost in the woods is a mystery. From later recon-
struction it appears that he went out the back door of his
house, which would have led him straight into the woods,
toward my house. The temperature outside was fairly
cold that morning — high 30's. Luckily, there wasn't much
snow on the ground that year.

Back at Mom's house, Jim had heard the door slam.
Mom was still asleep, so Jim went outside, knowing Dad
had probably left. Jim went to the front door, thinking it
the most logical door that Dad would go out. On seeing
no one, he got in the car, drove down the driveway and
went north down Wheeler Road. Of course, there were no
signs of Dad, who had gone the other way. Later Jim was
astonished to learn how far Dad had travelled in such a
short time, since he had gone out the door to start search-
ing as soon as he heard the door slam.

When I greeted my father at the door by hugging him,
as I normally would have, he did not respond in his usual
way. When I encouraged him to sit down, he paced and
acted as if he were leaving. I was worried that he would
leave and not know where to go.

"How about some breakfast, Pa?" I said, trying to
sound as normal as possible. "There might be poison in
it," he replied, very matter-of-factly, as if I should know
that to be the case. I suggested breakfast again and again,
but he refused to sit down or eat anything. "They're trying
to poison me," he said, pleadingly. I called Jim as soon
as I could and told him where Dad was. Jim said he would
come over as quickly as he could. I had all I could do to
keep my father in the house. He was so agitated and
confused, nothing he did would have surprised me.

He seemed to sense the need for help. His requests for
the sheriff seemed really to be cries for help from one who
knew what was happening to him. But the paranoia was
difficult to deal with. Here was a man whom I had become

much closer to over the last several years, whom I thought I knew very well, telling me he wouldn't eat anything I had to offer or even drink juice because they might be poisoned. Knowing that arguing had never worked with him, I remained calm, reassuring, and tried to calm him down, too. I'm not sure he knew who I was. Yet he had chosen my house to come to.

By now Jim had arrived. I went in the other room and called our local family physician, to whom I described the behavior and asked for guidance. He said he would have to return my call shortly after consulting with someone and reviewing the medication history I had provided. Jim kept Dad occupied in the kitchen as I talked on the phone in my office.

The next several moments dragged as we waited for some word of assistance to deal with this bewildered man sitting in the kitchen. The doctor called back and recommended a visit to a psychiatrist in Traverse City. Immediately I called her office and explained what had happened. She agreed to see him on her lunch hour at 12:00.

It was now about 9:00 a.m. We had a few hours to get Dad back home, dress him in more appropriate clothing, and drive to Traverse City. I called Ron, a family friend who lived next door to my folks, and told him the situation in case he was available to help. He came to their house and greeted Dad. Later he described Dad as "frantic, frightened, his eyes sunk in." After talking to him a few minutes, Ron convinced him to sit down and meditate. Even if he wasn't really meditating, he sat down and shut his eyes for 10 to 15 minutes. Afterward, refreshed, he appeared cognizant of his surroundings and briefly talked coherently for a few minutes.

Knowing that we had some extra time, Ron asked Dad if he wanted to take a walk to Ron's house. Dad complied, and they walked to the road. My parents had sold two acres to Ron about six months before. Dad remembered the sale. Now, as they came toward Ron's place, Dad put his arm around Ron, walked past the house, and said, "Do you want more land than this? Do you need any more land? Would you like another five or ten acres?"

Ron politely said, "No, thank you."

"If you need more land," Pa reiterated," you let me know."

A few hundred yards and some small talk later, Dad inquired, "How much land do you have?"

Ron answered, "This is a real beautiful two acres."

Dad looked blankly at him and said, "This is the biggest two acres I've ever seen in my life. This is more like five acres."

"No, John," Ron said sadly. "It's only two."

With no warning, my father's paranoia had returned. As he had always phrased it, he thought Ron was "against" him. After walking back to his own house, Dad got in his car with Ron's help. Jim and I drove him to the doctor's office in Traverse City. Mother was relieved. Jim was sad. I was afraid. My father was oblivious.

CHAPTER VII - Diagnosis

My father seemed to realize, at least briefly, that we were on our way for help. He said little during the 25-mile ride to the doctor's office. We weren't getting the sheriff, as he had requested, but there was relief in leaving the house in which he thought he was an intruder. After a brief consultation, the psychiatrist suggested that he be admitted to the psychiatric unit of the local medical center for observation and tests. Called Center One, this wing cares for patients with mental disorders, but is small and pleasant with brightly colored rooms, recreation and dining facilities, and a caring staff. It is an interim care setting for diagnosis and limited treatment. The maximum stay is about two weeks.

When my father was admitted, he was still wearing two layers of clothing and a heavy winter coat. The task of removing any of his clothes before admission had proved too difficult. We had left him the way he had appeared on my doorstep.

The admitting diagnosis on the hospital record was "arteriosclerotic vascular disease and depression" with an impression of "senile dementia" — a vague summary. Perhaps more tests would shed new light. We felt relieved. Maybe now we would find out what was wrong.

After getting him settled in his room, we returned to my mother's house and let her know what had happened.

She appeared relieved, but exhausted. Since she didn't want to be alone, Jim and I stayed with her that night. During the evening, sadness enveloped me like a dark cloud. It occurred to me that my father might not be coming home again. I went outside by myself, looked around at the beautiful stars and clear night, at the grounds of my parents' peaceful country home, and cried for our loss. My mother had hoped that when she was recovered from her hip operation she would be able to bring her life's partner home again. I did not share her optimism.

Dad's demeanor for the two weeks in Center One was jovial and generally docile. He wandered unwittingly into other patients' rooms and became lost easily. Once he strayed from the floor and was found in another section of the hospital. He spit some of his medications into the toilet and left the water running for no reason. The nurses watched him closely.

He mentioned to one nurse that he had run out of the house the day before because someone was trying to shoot him. In the last few months he had expressed fear that my mother would "run around" with another man. The paranoia surrounding this subject was now becoming paramount in his mind. He mentioned the subject repeatedly to the doctor and nurses and told them that this man was taking his belongings while he was in the hospital. The convolutions of his now demented mind seemed to become more and more difficult to unravel.

One morning he called my mother at home. Painfully, she reassured him she wasn't running around on him. He continued telling the nurse about her going places and having a married man over all the time. Briefly he mentioned that the fellow's wife was his own daughter, but the family connection was becoming irrelevant. All that mattered was that his wife was hanging around with another man.

There were times when he thought he was home. When walking in the hallway, he had his rubber boots and felt liners on. When asked whether these weren't too hot for indoor attire, he replied, "I might have to go to the garage, and I'll get my feet wet." One time he said he was looking for tools under the bed. Other times he would be looking for his father, who had been dead for more than 35 years.

He searched for my mother in the hallway and in other patients' rooms. He walked in and said, "How is my wife?" When he continually had trouble finding his room, the staff put a sign on his door with the word "JOHN" in foot-high letters. Sometimes the sign helped.

Despite his troubled fantasies about Mother and his frustration at not being able to remember names, he was jovial with the staff and appreciative of the care they gave him. When the psychiatrist finished talking to him for the day and started to leave the room, he followed her and said, "I'm not done yet. Listen to this one. I've got a good one for you," as if telling another joke. Sometimes she sat and listened to "one more," even though it made little sense.

One who listened well was my brother Paul. He came to see Dad a few days after admission. Paul remembers his trying to tell the events of the past few days — going to an unfamiliar house, being afraid the owner was going to come home, seeing another man in the house. The account didn't make much sense, but Paul understood some of it and could see the desperation behind it. Dad clearly knew Paul and found comfort in his ability to listen. Seeing a fresh face different from the characters he had been dealing with was welcome.

My father received a lot of attention on this ward, including attempts by the staff to play Yahtzee with him. He had always enjoyed this simple dice game, but now he couldn't even follow the instructions necessary for play. Yet one day my mother, Jim and I took him for a walk and ended up in the recreation room. There were a piano, some comfortable seats, and a Ping-Pong table. I suggested playing the piano and singing, but he made a gesture that he wanted to play Ping-Pong, an activity he rarely engaged in. The paddles were on the table, but I had to obtain the balls from the desk. I went quickly for fear his enthusiasm would wane.

He played Ping-Pong as well as he had done badly at Yahtzee. It was as if his motor skills would outlast his mental capacity for remembering number games. This man, who had rarely played Ping-Pong in his life, deftly hit the ball with spin and finesse. I played and watched at the same time, amazed at the step back in time we seemed to be taking. He laughed and even said a few things, and his otherwise self-conscious attitude temporarily disappeared. We were having pure unadulterated fun, which we rarely ever had together. The incident is etched in my memory, especially his smile. The smile was all there was that day. For a brief moment all was well. A few times he walked to another part of the room, but for the most part he focused on the playing. Suddenly, by leaving us and wandering into the hallway, he stopped the activity as quickly as he had started. He had played for 20 to 30 minutes, and now it was time to leave.

A few days later he had a consultation with a neurologist. Upon entering my father's room, the doctor noted that he was lying fully clothed in the bed and needed almost a minute to disentangle himself from the bedspread. He told the doctor his name was "John Dechow," but said his middle name was "Viola." His identification with my mother was complete. He was able to comply with some simple commands, but when asked to point to his left knee, he indicated instead the little finger on his left hand. When asked what a triangle is, he said, "It shows an intelligent person which way to go."

Later, the psychiatrist called us in to a comfortable meeting room to discuss my father's condition. She had consulted with the neurologist, who said in his report that the likelihood of Alzheimer's disease should be considered. She related that the diagnosis could not be determined definitely until after death, but that all signs pointed to Alzheimer's.

I had heard of the disease for the first time the previous fall and thought that possibly my father had it but now the words carried a certain finality. She explained the stages and said it appeared that his condition was advanced, but that a patient could suffer from Alzheimer's for anywhere from five to fifteen years after its onset. Mother, Paul, and I were present at this meeting. Questions bombarded the doctor like darts at a dartboard.

Perhaps she mentioned characteristics of the final stage. If she did, I don't remember. I wasn't ready to hear all the unpleasant details. I was ready for someone to tell us what to do, how to go on interacting with this man who sometimes knew us and sometimes didn't, how to tell him that he had to go to a foster care home and be cared for by someone else, since we couldn't handle him. She suggested a foster care home, because it appeared that minimal restrictions were called for and a nursing home wasn't necessary as yet. He could stay in the hospital up to two weeks so we could have time to find an appropriate placement.

I went home that night and thought about what the doctor had said. Did she say there was no cure? I thought so. He could last five to fifteen years from the onset? How would we handle it? How would my mother live? How could she pay for nursing home care? Would he have good days and then dwindle further and further into a yet unforeseen demented state? What would the end be like? How long would he be able to remain in foster care? Would he understand that we loved him and were trying to do the best we could for him? The questions exploded in my mind. I couldn't sleep. I tried to remember my father of years past. The images were comforting, but right now they were much weaker than the vision of a man shuffling his feet and looking for my mother in the hallway. Tomorrow we would do what we had to do — choose his next home.

CHAPTER VIII - Foster Care

"Why is that gate across the doorway?" I asked. Matter-of-factly, the woman replied, "Oh, we can't have them coming in the kitchen while we're trying to cook dinner. We don't leave it up all the time." What she said sounded reasonable, but I wondered to myself, "What if they have to stay in that room for hours at a time?"

The-eight-by-twenty-four-foot room was pleasant enough, with large windows, a color TV, a card table and comfortable chairs. There were about eight to ten people. Some were nodding off to sleep. Others were watching TV or were sitting and staring out the window, waiting for supper or just waiting. They were mostly old—many heads of white hair, many feeble bones trying to move, somewhat unsuccessfully, from chair to sofa or sofa to window or aimlessly from one side of the room to the other.

Dinner would be in about an hour. The foster care home operator was supervising a couple of people who were preparing dinner in the large kitchen for the 10 to 12 residents. Paul and I had appointments that day to look at a couple other such homes in order to find one for our father to stay in. From the Department of Social Services I had learned the procedures and costs involved in placing someone in foster care and the names of at least eight foster care homes in our county and the next that might have openings. I called them all. I had narrowed the list down to three due to the fact that some were now full, some refused to take Alzheimer's patients, and some were too far away. The average cost, I discovered, was between six and eight hundred dollars per month. This usually included trips to the doctor or hospital and a couple outings a month in addition to food, shelter, and general caretaking.

The home we were now seeing was a large and pleasant one, but was located on a major highway 20 miles away. I imagined my father strolling out of the house onto the highway, either being hit by a car or wandering aimlessly. The woman who showed us the place reassured us that in their 10 to 15 years of caring for people only one man had gotten out of the house, and he had been picked up by the sheriff shortly after he had left.

The woman took us up a long flight of stairs to a back bedroom, the one available for Dad. The room was small, but clean and pleasant. I noticed down a hallway an outside stairway, probably necessary in case of fire, and I asked the woman how easily a person could get out. She stated that the door to the stairs was always locked and would not be easy to open. I remembered my dad's persistence and hoped there was a better alternative to this home.

The next place was small. I couldn't imagine how it had become licensed. The five or six residents were sitting in the living room. The TV was on, but no one seemed to be watching. They stared blankly until someone said something. Then a brief conversation would ensue. The operator of this home seemed anxious for us to take the available room. She enthusiastically explained their delicious menus, their outings for the patients, the fun they had, and how they related as a family. The house was located on a less travelled road than the first. But it was still 20 miles from my home, and its individual rooms were small, dark, and depressing. Paul mentioned to me that the menus the caretaker had described sounded unrealistic. He said he didn't eat as well as she was describing and he had more money to work with than the home's limited budget. We went home discouraged.

The next day we went to see the third and last home on the list. Closer to my home by about five miles than the other two, this one was a large secluded farmhouse in the country. Its location on a little used gravel road was appealing. The couple who ran it were young and energetic and said they had handled Alzheimer's patients before. The room available was a double, and Dad would be sharing it with another gentleman about whose problems we didn't inquire.

Four children were in the home too, whose youth might serve to enliven the place. The rooms were large, cheery, and nicely furnished. An orchard and barn were in the back. My instincts told me that this was the one to choose above the others, because the people were more genuinely friendly and caring. Paul did not share my enthusiasm, but agreed that this was the best pick of the three.

We told Mother of our findings, and she agreed to this last home. We took care of the necessary arrangements and let the people know we could bring our father as soon as his release, which would be on Wednesday, April 13.

On Wednesday afternoon we went to the hospital to take him to his new home. But first there were financial matters to attend to.

The only piece of property still in his name alone was my parents' 1977 Chevy. We had transferred a bank account from his name to Mom's and Dad's the week before when he seemed lucid enough to write his name and understand what we were doing. Afraid the day was quickly coming that he would not understand any piece of paper or transaction placed in front of him, we thought it best to make one last transfer. I had brought the car title with me. I made arrangements with the nurse, who told us we could use the activity room.

I walked into Dad's room to get him, not knowing what to expect. I told him we needed to sign some papers and asked him to come down the hall with me to another room. Paul, Mother, Father, and I went into a room with a large table where we all sat down. He actually remained seated long enough for me to explain that it would be good if he signed the title for the 1977 Chevy so my mother could take care of it. He made a gesture as if he understood. I showed him where to sign and he did so, thereby giving up the last hold he had on anything by himself.

He didn't protest, as he would have in the past over such an action, and yet I was sure he understood what was happening. He nodded his head up and down as if approving, but his face was solemn and downcast. On some level he knew he was unable to conduct his own affairs. Perhaps he was relieved that someone else could take over. I was relieved that the chore was done, but sad that this step had to be taken.

The signing complete, he was ready to get up. He had been given a sedative for the trip ahead, so that we wouldn't find ourselves unable to control him. He acted relatively quiet. We told him we were taking him to a foster care home, because Mother had to have her hip operated on. We told him the home was in the country near Lake Leelanau and we thought he would like it. He said little on the way out, but seemed anxious to leave the hospital and ride in the car.

The car ride to the home was uneventful. He appeared to be heavily sedated. I looked at what my father had become and thought, *"Is this what I can look forward to as I grow old? If so, let me die first."*

We arrived at a picturesque home in the midst of fruit farms and helped him out of the car. He asked where we were, and I said he would be staying here for a while. Mother told him she had to have her hip operated on, she would be unable to care for him right now, and he would get good care here. He gave us a blank stare and immediately started walking aimlessly. We introduced him to Doug and Sue (not their real names), and they showed us to his room. It was a cheerful room with the sun shining through the window onto the bed. There were two single beds, and a dresser and chair for each occupant.

We brought his suitcase in with us and started emptying his belongings into the dresser. Sue said she would do that later, we didn't have to bother, but we were not ready to leave and wanted to busy ourselves with his clothes.

Paul and Doug kept him busy while my mother and I handled the financial arrangements with Sue. When we completed the transaction, both Doug and Sue advised that it would be better if we did not visit him for a week to ten days, so that his adjustment would be smoother. From their experience they had learned that patients adjust to their new surroundings easier if they don't see family members for a number of days. Mom and I said we understood and would comply with their request. However, Paul was returning to Ann Arbor in a few days, and he would like to see Dad again before leaving and would be back.

Doug and Sue had four children. With them, my father thought he was back in school. When they went outside to play, he went along and tried to supervise them. He called to them and said, "Come on, children. It's time to come in now." He referred to school constantly and made sense for a change when he spoke of it. Only occasionally, when his mind strayed to another subject, would he lose coherence.

He went out with them when they waited for the school bus. He played with them outside when they returned home. He chased them around the house and beckoned to them, "Come on, children. Come on." He clapped his hands and told them school was about to start. Rather than fearing him or treating him as a mental patient, as some adults would have, the children enjoyed the game and encouraged his play with them.

Inside, Dad did things, he said, to protect the children. He took knives out of drawers and, when asked what he was doing, said he was afraid the kids would be hurt and was moving the knives to a safer place.

Then he started moving furniture. He seemed to think that if he moved everything out of the way nobody would fall and get hurt. He took the lamp from the bedroom and put it in the toilet tank. He put his clothes in the stool. He put the bathroom scales in the sink, ripped the curtains off the window, took the drawers out of his dresser, and pulled his mattress partially onto the floor. When Sue or Doug noticed his behavior, one of them asked, "Why are you doing this, John?" He replied something about school and being a teacher.

Once at mealtime he sat down to eat. But the minute Sue turned around to get another plate, he was up and walking. He generally couldn't sit still for more than a minute or two unless someone stood right near him and prevented his leaving. To Sue he seemed confused the first day, then became more and more agitated the second and third days. He constantly fidgeted with anything within reach. He put the button of his shirt in his hand and played with it. Then all of a sudden he ripped it off. After the scissors he had found were taken away, he ripped up his clothes with his bare hands, not maliciously, but as if such an act were the thing to do.

Sue and Doug said he appeared heavily medicated when he arrived. When he didn't seem to be calming down, they called the doctor, who changed his medication. Only two days into his stay he became even more agitated. He wandered around all day, couldn't sit still, and much to their dismay he continued this behavior into the night. He couldn't sleep, and neither could they for having to be on alert for his wanderings.

They started taking shifts watching him at night so one at least could get some sleep. His mind was fighting sleep, and he wasn't about to succumb to the needs of his body. He had been through many changes in the past two weeks — too many for his addled brain to cope with. In the course of his four-day stay at the foster care home, it's doubtful that he slept more than one hour.

He still dressed himself. The only trouble was that he did it over and over again, donning his pajamas, then long underwear, a flannel shirt, a heavy jacket, two pairs of pants, and his shoes on the wrong feet. He snapped his glasses in two so he wouldn't have to worry about them anymore.

Occasionally he mentioned Mother and her need for an operation, as if he understood. At other times he would look down at the floor, shake his head, and say, "I can't remember anymore." A meeting long ago at school he tried to remember. He even asked Sue to call a certain individual to make sure he was going to be present. As if to snap himself back to reality, he looked down again and said, "I'm not the way I used to be." The awareness, however, was momentary. A moment later he'd be walking down the hall, shuffling his feet, a blank look in his eye, in search of his memory in a torn curtain.

By Saturday night, only four days after he had arrived, he was weaving like a drunk, staggering, and often falling. He was tearing his sheets and clothes more than before, and once Doug had to hold him down when he started kicking. The more tired he was, the more aggravated he became. He still went to the bathroom if you physically led him, sat him down, and waited. Once, while Doug was with him in the bathroom, holding his shoulders and telling him to go, he tried unsuccessfully to hit Doug, but was too weak. Doug stopped him and said, "Now, John, you don't want to do that." Dad responded, "Yeah, you're right. I don't want to do that." He stopped the erratic behavior as quickly as he had started it.

Doug and Sue found it difficult to stay angry at him, because he would apologize for his behavior. In the midst of one of his wanderings Sue requested, "John, will you please sit down? You're going to get hurt." He sat down, looking like a guilty child with chocolate smears on his face, and said, "I'm sorry."

On Sunday morning Doug and Sue made a difficult decision. They had tried to phone us the night before, but we had not been home. They felt that they could not care for him anymore. He had fallen once again, but this time on an antique table, and had crushed it flat. More important than the value of the table was the fact that he could hurt himself or someone else with his staggering and falling. As foster care homes are not allowed to restrain patients, the choice to send him elsewhere was not one of comfort, but of safety.

Doug called the doctor to see if Dad could be readmitted to the same unit he had been released from, but the doctor was unavailable. The unit had no bed available anyway. Doug called the sheriff's department and was advised to phone the local state psychiatric hospital. When he did so, the doctor was to return his call. But after more than an hour with no response, Doug felt he had waited long enough. He and his 16-year-old son got Dad into a truck, seated between them, and drove him the 20 miles to the hospital. With his seat belt on and unable to get up, Dad was accommodating. He fell asleep a few times during the trip, after discovering that his attempts at standing were futile.

When they arrived at the state hospital, a large local psychiatric hospital, they were made to wait and wait and wait. They were there for three to four hours, because this was to be an involuntary admission, which was tantamount to having someone committed. Once again, we were not available and had no idea all of this was transpiring. I don't know what we would have done had we known.

At first the admitting people Doug talked to said they couldn't take Dad without a doctor's order. They then tried to find his doctor, but were unsuccessful. Doug said he would not take my father home and was leaving him there because "he's dangerous to himself and others." As Doug put it, "Everybody in the house is on the ragged edge." Finally, Doug was told he would have to sign the patient in himself. When he got up to do so and stopped watching Dad for a brief moment, Dad was up and bouncing down the hallway, oblivious to what was transpiring.

The deed was done. At 6:00 p.m. on Sunday, April 17, 1983, my father became an involuntary admission to a psychiatric hospital.

CHAPTER IX - Court

I knew what my mother was thinking as she and I walked up the steps of the yellowing old building, the registration office of the state hospital, to learn my dad's ward and room number, so we could visit him. We almost said the words at the same time. "I never thought we'd be coming to visit him here."

Her father had died in this hospital after many lonely years of confinement. Her sister, too, was still a patient here, after having been in and out of the place for more than 30 years. Many times my mother had walked the halls on the way to visit one or the other of them and had heard the screams and ravings of those who inhabited its decrepit old rooms. Only recently had I started to visit my aunt, but I knew, though to a lesser extent, the fear and anguish my mother felt.

At least here we wouldn't need to worry about Dad wandering into the street or even off the floor he was on. He was under lock and key. I went to the desk and said expectantly, "Lynn McAndrews and Viola Dechow to see John Dechow." The clerk directed us to the floor he was on and said, "Knock loudly on the door, so the guard will hear you. I'll let them know you're coming. Just follow the blue lines on the wall."

Some of the hallways were poorly lit, as was the entrance to the elevator that would take us to our destination. The quiet of the halls was eerie. Office hours were over, and the skeleton crew was maintaining the workings of the behemoth institution.

We arrived at the heavy metal door leading to my father's floor. It had a small rectangular window in the upper portion with metal strips across it. The door was locked securely. I knocked as hard as I could. My mother waited in the wings leaning on her walker, appearing forlorn and tired.

The attendant finally came to the door, opened it, and invited us inside. I asked him where my father was. He said he would find out if Dad was in his own room or in one of the common rooms. The attendant disappeared into a room, returned, and indicated where to go. I discovered later we had visited my father in the "time-out room," named for patients who were giving others a hard time.

The room was large and antiseptic-looking. It had bare floors, barred windows, and no furniture except the one chair my dad was sitting in. It was a "geri-chair," a large, comfortable, padded chair with a tray across the front allowing one to be restrained. On visits to local nursing homes I had seen many of these lately, and the patients tied in them— an apparently necessary evil when the patient-caretaker ratio is sometimes ten to one.

The male nurse said he would find some chairs for us to sit in. When we entered the room, my father did not look up. He was dressed in one of his own shirts and pants, and his white hair was disheveled. As we got close to him, he seemed to notice that someone was in the room. He looked up at us and stared blankly. I said, "Hi, Pa. It's Lynn and Ma. How are you?" With no response, no smile, he returned his gaze to the tray table in front of him. He was touching every spot on the table as if it were giving him some pleasurable sensation each time he moved his fingers. Over and over again he rubbed an imaginary object, then rubbed his thumb against his other fingers, as if touching them for the first time. He ran his fingers around the edge of the table, under it, then on the top once again. I thought, "*Who is this man? He can't be my father.*" However confused he had seemed before, his appearance shocked me.

This was the first time I had seen my father this powerless and helpless, restrained. His cheeks were sunken, and he showed no sign that he recognized either of us. When the nurse returned with a few chairs, I asked if I could take my father in the hallway to see if he wanted to walk. The nurse agreed. I started taking Dad's restraint off. He looked askance at me for a moment, then, realizing he could get up, did so. He began to walk. The steps he took were small and shuffling. My mother sat down, and I told her we would return shortly.

We walked into the hallway, and I watched as my father walked along the walls with side railings, holding onto them, touching them as thoroughly as he had the tray table moments before. He arrived at the locked door and touched the doorknob, going over it thoroughly with his fingers. He didn't act as if he wanted to open the door, only to touch it, as if making an imprint of its substance on his fingers. I repeated to him who I was and again inquired about his welfare. He didn't respond, but only relished in his tactile sense on yet another wall, railing, or piece of door hardware.

The nurse had been in and out of an office 30 to 40 feet down the hall for the few minutes Dad had been walking, perhaps keeping an eye on us. When the nurse reappeared, I asked if he would help me put Dad back in his chair so Mom could attempt to talk to him. We took him by the arm and led him back to the chair in the bare room. Dad didn't protest.

The nurse said, "John, don't you want to visit with your wife and daughter?"

"Yes. Where are they?" he replied. When we again showed him where and who we were, he half smiled and went right back to fidgeting with the tray table.

I asked my mother if she would mind being alone for a few minutes while I went to talk to the nurse. She hesitated, then asked what she should do. I could see the fear in her eyes. She didn't want to be left alone with him. I assured her that he was securely tied in and suggested that she try holding his hand. I had taken his hand a few times. It was warm and strong and I enjoyed holding it, even though I knew he would rather be exploring his tray table.

I talked to the nurse for several minutes, inquiring about my father's condition. Was he eating? Did he sleep all night? Was he incontinent? What drugs was he on? The nurse willingly answered all my questions, then gave me my father's watch and what was left of his glasses. Without them Dad's confusion was accentuated, as he wore his glasses often and would have difficulty seeing. I took his belongings reluctantly, unwilling to admit fully he wouldn't or couldn't make use of these items again. The nurse stated that I would have to talk to the doctor or hospital social worker for more detailed information on his prognosis or on his future. I said I would do so. The thought foremost in my mind was, *"How do I get my father out of here?"*

Several phone calls later (to the doctor, hospital social worker, probate court worker, Social Services worker), I discovered that we were almost in a Catch 22 situation. Since my father had been admitted involuntarily, we could not obtain his release merely by signing a piece of paper. A hearing would have to be scheduled in Probate Court. A mental health investigator would have to assess my father's condition. Unless an alternative plan were offered, he would most likely be ordered to stay at the psychiatric hospital indefinitely. To add to the urgency, whatever funds my parents had saved would quickly diminish in light of the fact that the ward he was on cost $200 per day, $6,000 per month. No insurance would pay for his care there, including Medicare, since the hospital was in a state of flux and was currently not certified.

Even though the doctor at the hospital advised against quick release, saying my father needed more than a week to ten days to "stabilize," I explained the situation to the Probate Court worker and pleaded for as early a hearing date as possible. It was set for Monday, April 25, at 9:15 a.m.

Meanwhile, I hoped I could find a nursing home that would take him in his current condition—an Alzheimer's patient who was occasionally uncooperative and belligerent. Luckily, I had already visited some of the nearby nursing homes, so I wasn't starting from scratch. To my disappointment, the one closest to home did not have any openings, so I had to deal with the larger ones in Traverse City, none of which was my first choice. I found one in a lower price range that had an opening, had dealt with Alzheimer's patients for a while, and had several of them currently. The admissions person said the home could take my father at any time. I said we would be in touch pending the outcome of the court hearing.

The court mental health investigator even researched a few nursing homes that were three hours away, but had greater expertise in dealing with my father's problem. I discouraged this possibility, as we wanted him as close to home as possible.

About this time in my discovery of the bureaucracy surrounding the elderly, health care, and social service institutions, I learned how difficult the financial situation could be for an older person with health problems. My parents' entire savings could be wiped out in less than two years with payments to the state hospital and to foster care and to nursing homes. I learned that, if a person needs "basic care" in a nursing home, i.e., custodial care, and no "skilled nursing" is required, then Medicare or private insurance will not pay anything. Social Services cannot help unless the victim's resources have dwindled to $3,000 and the spouse's to $10,000 in addition to their house and personal belongings. (This may vary from state to state, and the figures may have changed slightly since 1983.)

Then there was the added burden of legal guardianship if one had not had the foresight to have the afflicted person sign over property or accounts while still able to do so.

I saw my father a few more times before his hearing on the 25th. He was just as non-responsive to me as the first time and appeared frail and much older than his 72 years. The doctor had suggested that he be taken off all drugs for a few days to stabilize him. When I saw him the second time, he didn't act as wired and anxious as he had a few days earlier. His psychiatrist from the medical hospital had continued efforts at getting him admitted to that place, but there was no room. Now that he was an involuntary admission, moving him would require a court hearing anyway.

I desperately wanted my father out of the state hospital after hearing through the grapevine that a social worker's father, who had been a patient for several years, had been near death for several months in the final stages of Alzheimer's. He could no longer swallow and was totally bedridden. Oblivious to his own state, he was fed nutrients by tubes. Tubes also collected his waste, and he had to be turned over every half hour. My father's progression might not be any faster in another environment, but we as his family might at least be able to choose more wisely about IV feeding and about prolonging his life by artificial means.

During the remainder of my father's stay in the state hospital, he displayed more of the same behavior that we had seen before. He continued to wander. Left in an unlocked room, he interfered with painters on the ward and got into fresh paint. He took toilet paper holders down and tried to dress himself by putting his pillowcase on his feet.

Sometimes at meals he could figure out how to use his eating utensils. Other times he had to be spoon fed. The patients were given a time in the afternoon when they were allowed to smoke. Dad requested a cigarette, even though he hadn't smoked for about 35 years. When the aide gave him one, he didn't know how to hold it to get a light.

Even though he slept better on some nights, on others he was awake all night and wandered about. Once he slept in the geri chair all night. On another night he was poseyed in his bed — side rails were up and a vest restricted him — yet somehow he managed to get out of the bed. On still another night he was found nude, while tearing sheets from the bed. He strongly resisted the nurse's attempt to return him to bed.

The wandering and restless behavior of Alzheimer's patients after dark is so common that it has been given a name: "sundowner syndrome." This is the patient's way of fighting something he or she doesn't understand and indicates his or her confusion about who or where they are.

Although my father's medications had been stopped when he first arrived at the state hospital, many different drugs were later used to treat the sleep difficulty, the agitation, the restlessness, and the disruptive behavior: Vistaril, Haldol, Cogentin, Benadryl, Halcion, and Dalmane. The change in his behavior was minimal.

On Monday, April 25, 1983, my mother, Jim, and I drove the 12 miles to the courthouse, mostly in silence. I did not fear what would happen at the hearing, since everyone I had spoken to about its outcome had been supportive and cooperative. Rather, I feared what my father would look like and how he would act if brought to the hearing. Would he recognize us? I didn't know what to expect as we walked up the steps of the courthouse, sat in the courtroom, and waited. Would he be brought to this proceeding? Was it necessary to subject him to yet another insult? Since the deputy was late bringing him to the courtroom, I had what seemed an interminable number of minutes to contemplate these questions.

The hospital's record states that no drugs were given to my father that morning before he was taken to court. But when I saw him, my first thought was, *"They must have him all doped up, more so than usual, for the trip here."* He shuffled into the courtroom on the arm of the deputy and took a seat where he was directed. Head down, white hair uncombed, he appeared to stare at the floor. Unaware of his surroundings, he didn't look our way. More docile than I had ever seen him, he didn't try to wander or touch the table at which he sat. Instead, he sat with hands in his lap, nodding, nearly falling asleep. He was gaunt and his clothes hung on him like on a limp doll.

My attention turned from him when I heard the familiar, "All rise, Court is in session." I was glad for the momentary diversion. More quickly than expected, the hearing was over. It was actually a formality ordering what we had already agreed to outside. The judge presented the background of how my father came to be here and of the alternative treatment plan we had worked out — placement in a nursing home instead of remaining in the state hospital. Doug from the foster care home, who had no real interest in keeping us from doing what we preferred, did not attend the hearing.

After making sure we had no questions about the arrangement, the judge discharged my father via court order on a 90-day Alternative Treatment Order to the nursing home in Traverse City and/or to the local one if an opening became available. If the nursing home found that he was unable to cooperate, he would have to be returned to the state hospital and receive the maximum 60 days of treatment.

The hearing was over in less than 15 minutes. As a formality my father was asked if he understood or objected to the judgment. He looked at the floor and said nothing. He was unaware when the hearing was over and had to be led out of the courtroom. He was our responsibility now, and we took him from the deputy.

Finally, he looked at us. A faint smile creeped into his countenance, but he said nothing, only followed our lead as we walked to the car. We escorted him into the front seat, Mom to the back, and started the 25-plus mile drive to yet another new home. Emotionally exhausted from the continuing ordeal, I wondered how much longer those of us living with my father's struggle could continue.

Chapter X - Nursing Home

I compare the moving of my father to the transporting of a prisoner from one facility to another. We in his family didn't know what to expect from this man whom we thought we knew so well. Adding to our anxiety was the fact that we had to stop at the state hospital to obtain his "exit papers" so that the nursing home would know his medications, behavior, nutritional needs, and allergies. When the car stopped near the hospital entrance, he made no protest. In fact, the entire trip was almost as if he weren't there. He nodded occasionally as if falling asleep and was very docile. However annoying his questions of weeks past had been, I longed for one now, if only to show us some spirit remained. None came.

We obtained the papers and drove to the nursing home. I had visited this nursing home before, as I had just moved my mother's sister here from the state hospital a few weeks before. I had hoped this would not be a place in which I had to put anyone. But there was no choice in the matter since room was now available here, and not elsewhere. The nursing home seemed large, with capacity for up to 100 patients. Yet on some shifts there was only one aide for every 12 patients. When I managed to talk to an aide, he or she seemed overworked. Occasionally it would be difficult to find anyone to talk to in the hallway or in the patients' rooms.

The home was located on a country road just outside the city. The views from different directions varied — a mobile home park, an abandoned house, rolling fields stretching to the horizon. In the front were flowers and grass, a small decorative fence, lawn chairs, and a few outdoor tables. At the entrance to the building a small well-decorated lobby looked like a small living room where one could sit and talk to guests. The stench of urine would occasionally reach one's nostrils, but it wasn't overpowering, and at least there was carpeting instead of institutional type bare floors. The halls fanned out from the central nurse's station like spokes of a wheel, with the dining room and kitchen area closest to the nurse's station.

Plenty of help greeted our arrival. An attendant came to the car to help escort my father into the building. The administrator escorted my mother and me into her office while Jim went with Dad to my father's assigned room. The administrator explained that we would have to sign a few forms for the admission. They all seemed routine. The one that I was not prepared for was the Patient's Personal Effects Inventory. On a single sheet of paper was a list of the items my father still had in the world: two jackets, four shirts, eight pair of socks, five handkerchiefs, one comb, one belt, a pair of boots, three pairs of pajamas. Of course, we would bring him what he needed, and he had property left at home, but to him none of it mattered anymore. His material world was reduced to a small list, and even this he could no longer comprehend. He would walk from room to room giving away personal items or he would take those of others and later not remember where he put them or why he took them in the first place.

Having completed the paperwork, we went to the room where he was taken. The room was pleasant, colorful, open, very different from the atmosphere of the state hospital.

I looked at my father. The meticulous man I once knew was gone. His hair was disheveled, his beard had a few particles of food in it, his clothes were wrinkled and a stain appeared here and there. I remembered how he used to dress when we would go to church or out to dinner. His suit would be crisply pressed, everything in place, his tie neatly tied, shoes shined, pants creased just so. I used to love the way he smelled — from the Old Spice cologne he always wore. Now I noticed an odor about him that reeked of an unclean body. It was a body neglected by an owner who had self-respect no more, a man oblivious to the need for grooming and personal hygiene.

After a little while in my father's room, we stopped to see my aunt briefly to tell her that Dad was here. She hadn't seen him in a few years, but perhaps she would be able to communicate with him.

Once again, as at the other placements, the nurse advised that there would be an "adjustment period" for my father while he became accustomed to a new routine. As I walked out the door, I wondered why anyone would ever want to become accustomed to living in this place. Although less restricting to the patient than the state hospital, the noise level was higher and the privacy nonexistent. I heard patients yelling for a nurse and wondered why a nurse or aide did not come. Later I realized that the screams continued even when the nurse did as requested. For the staff to comply with every yell or request was physically impossible.

Nor was the setting ideal for an Alzheimer's patient who could easily become disoriented. Four hallways led from a central core, and occasionally even I went down the wrong one and walked one-third of the way to the end before realizing my error. A setting with 100-plus patients provided too many stimuli for an already confused person to sort out.

In the next five or six days my father flashed in and out of reality. He walked with assistance and was alert but confused. Occasionally he would refuse to eat. He tore his bed linen, was often incontinent, and had sudden mood changes from passive and gentle to violent and uncooperative.

When the social worker stopped in, Dad repeatedly asked for my mother. Then, when she came to visit, he appeared not to notice her.

That weekend I assisted in putting on a communications workshop, a powerful experience that contributed to my ability to just "be" with my father as he was, rather than expecting him to act a certain way or wishing he were some other way. Monday morning, after completing my duties and escorting the workshop leader to the airport, I went to see my father before returning home to work. The halls were relatively quiet in the mid-morning. Breakfast was long past, lunch in the future.

I walked into my father's room. What I saw jolted me. He was lying naked in the bed with no covers or sheet on him. The bed's side rails were up so that he could not get out. He was lying on his side, legs half curled up toward his torso, his body approaching the fetal position. His body was very thin, wrinkled — old. He was awake, but stared at the wall blankly. His hair was uncombed and saliva drooled from his mouth onto his beard and chin. This was my father at his most vulnerable. I had never seen him like this before.

I pulled the sheet up over his bare body and said, "Hello." He looked up at me and surprisingly greeted me with a familiar twinkle in his eye that I hadn't seen in a while. I began talking. He acted as if he understood. Then he made the old familiar statement that, "I can't remember things anymore. I don't know what's wrong with me." So I told him what was wrong with him. With the exception of my brother Paul, who had attempted to explain his disease to him at the foster care home, no one had explained Alzheimer's disease to my father. In general, he may no longer have been able to understand. Yet, at least in his lucid moments, he surely had a right to know. I said, "Pa, you have Alzheimer's disease. It's the reason you are losing your memory." He looked at me for a brief moment as if he understood and appreciated the knowledge. Then he changed the subject as if what I had said were irrelevant.

After talking a few more minutes, I found an aide to help put his clothes back on. As I left, I was hoping there would soon be an opening at the local nursing home. He needed constant supervision and didn't appear to be getting it where he was. I had put his name on the local home's waiting list a couple weeks before, but with room for only 25 patients the home had infrequent openings.

My mother and I had both told my father that she had to go to Ann Arbor for a hip replacement. Whatever part of him still understood we felt had a right to know. On Wednesday, May 4, we stopped to see him on our way to Ann Arbor. He didn't show outward signs of understanding when we told him where we were going, but later I got reports that he had been exceptionally restless that night, had somehow managed to remove himself from the restraints of his geri chair without anyone's notice, and was caught walking in the hallway. When an orderly tried to take him back to his room and chair, Dad started hitting him hard.

My mother's operation was on Friday that week. I stayed in Ann Arbor through part of Sunday, which was Mother's Day. I remember sitting in the waiting room of the hospital while she was in the operating room and thinking, *"What will be will be, but please don't let anything happen to her now, not while Pa is in such bad shape."* I didn't know how I would handle another trauma right now.

I returned home and stopped to see my father on the way. I told him the operation had gone well and that Mom would be staying with Paul and Joanne for three or four weeks to recuperate. He acted as if he partly understood. I wondered what he would be saying if he comprehended fully. I wondered what he thought, in those moments when he was lucid, about being in this place. I wondered how tormented he felt when he realized his memory loss. My only consolation was the knowledge that those moments would not last much longer.

A few days later, on Wednesday, May 11, a program on Alzheimer's was given at a local senior center. A doctor talked about the disease — the progress on its cure and diagnosis, how to handle loved ones who had it, general information. I learned that one out of six people in the United States will contract the disease, that it is the fourth leading cause of death after heart disease, cancer, and stroke, that there is no cure and no remission, that a few people get it in their thirties, and that it can last from five to fifteen years.

One out of six? Could this be the way I go? Is it hereditary? Is there any prevention? Why me? I had more questions than there were answers. From then on I sought out as much information as I could and tried to educate others. I was surprised to learn how many people had not yet heard of this killer.

After learning what I already sensed, that a smaller setting is better for Alzheimer's patients, I was relieved when the local nursing home called and said it now had room for my father. I arranged with my dad's sister and her husband to drive with me when I picked him up, since I wasn't sure that he wouldn't try to get out of the car. They agreed to help, although I know it was difficult for my aunt to see her brother as he had become.

When I went in to get him once again I had to sign a form regarding his personal belongings. What I signed for was two pair of pants and four pair of socks, just a small part of what had been brought in with him. When I asked about his other belongings, the nurse said they were probably in the laundry and asked if I could come back in a few days to get the rest. I said I would and we left.

The 20-mile ride to the other nursing home was long. Once again, Dad asked if we shouldn't be turning at several roads we passed. My uncle, who was driving, remained calm and gave assurance that we were going the right way. The sun was shining. The day was beautiful. An unknowing observer could have seen us as a family just out for a drive in the country.

Chapter XI - Final Home

The sun shone in through the window and filled the room with afternoon light. We stood in a circle at the end of the hospital bed. There were six of us: myself, my aunt and uncle, the nurse and nurse's aide, and my dad. For the moment my father was the center of attention, smiling and making introductions. Were it not for his attire, his disheveled appearance, and the non sequiturs coming from his mouth, he could have been mistaken for the activities director of the nursing home.

He introduced his sister by name to the nurse, no easy task for him. We were all pleased at his momentary recall, especially my aunt, who experienced much pain in witnessing his erratic behavior. It was as if he were gathering us around him to give us instructions, for he started pointing out to each one of us where to sit or stand in the room. Most of what he said made little sense, but he was making an effort and smiling, and for this I was grateful.

Later, when it became apparent that his attention was waning, we decided to leave and let him become accustomed to his new home. The trip had been without incident. He had recognized his sister and called her by name. He had acted pleasant. What more could one ask?

We had moved him on May 12. My mother did not return from Ann Arbor until June 18. Her operation had been successful, but she needed time with Paul and Joanne to recuperate before returning home. I went to see my father a few times a week and encouraged whoever I could to visit him.

His first few weeks were a period of adjustment. For his own safety, he often needed the bed belts — two cotton ties strapped across his chest and hips to the sides of the bed. After he was allowed to walk for a while, he didn't even object to the belt being placed on him. Belligerent at times, he might swing at the nurses or aides, but was generally docile. He sometimes played with his food, poured milk into his Jello, threw his dishes or food on the floor, and started another strange habit of spitting on the floor. As if he were a child again, he talked to the nurses about going to "Grandma and Grandpa's house" and about asking "Momma to help us."

I wondered if his occasional more violent behavior related to visits from family members. I visited him on Sunday, June 12. The weather was warm outside. I took him out and walked with him around the grounds of the home. The greenery and flowers were appealing and the sound of birds chirping filled the air. I helped guide him around as one would a horse in a training ring. He didn't object at the first turn, but then later wanted to turn another way, toward the road. This inclination I discouraged quickly. I said, "Listen, Pa. Do you hear the bird singing?" He stopped, cocked his head to one side, said nothing, then continued walking. Could it be he understood and enjoyed? I hoped so.

Walking with him was satisfying. He said little, smiled occasionally, looked at me as if trying to figure out who I was and why I was there. But I loved him anyway, and his response to my caring, right now, didn't matter. We stayed outside for a while. When we went back inside, the nurse informed me that he had missed his "bathroom time." They found that if they took him at a certain time every day, he would cooperate and not go in his clothes. When the schedule was disrupted, however, his response was to act as a child by wetting his pants. I discovered later that after I left he not only soiled his pants, but also tore up the curtain divider and wall board and took his clothes off. Were his actions in reaction to my visits or to the fact that he had missed his potty break? The weekend of June 18 I drove to Ann Arbor to pick up my mother. Although very sad about my father's present condition, my mother was experiencing a great deal of freedom by having him out of the home. She purchased some items in Ann Arbor that she could never have bought when he was home. Either he didn't want her to have them, or else she was so tied to caring for him that she had no chance to shop. We returned from Ann Arbor with a U-Haul filled with a new living room sofa-bed, a dryer, and a dishwasher — items she had been wanting for some years. As soon as we got near her house, we stopped at the nursing home and saw Dad. My mother was still using a walker occasionally, as she would for a while, and was slow in entering the nursing home. On the trip we had discussed what had happened — the move from one home to the other and the details of his behavior. Her absence from him had improved her peace of mind. Now she was ready to see him again.

We walked slowly into his room. He was sitting in his chair. I said, "Pa, look who's here to see you." He looked up and smiled. His attention stayed with Mom for quite a while. We explained to him what had happened to her and hoped he understood. She needed comfort now as much as he did. Unfortunately, it would not be coming from him. Like a child, he took his own needs as paramount.

His beard, I thought, gave him a distinguished look. It was all white and full, and it matched his now all white hair. However, it was difficult to keep clean. Those who cared for him requested that they be allowed to shave it off. My mother assented, and he was once more clean shaven. He appeared even more gaunt than before. Long before his illness our family had planned a 50th anniversary party for my parents to be held at a local townhall on July 10. Coming for the reunion celebration would be family members from Florida and California, including six granddaughters and my brothers and sister. Also, my parents' many friends and local relatives had been invited. Although my father had to enter the nursing home, we decided to go ahead with the party, whether or not he could attend.

My father's absence cast a pall over the 50th anniversary celebration. Sixty or seventy people were there to wish my mother well, and she had a great time seeing relatives and friends. I had even thought of renting a band, since my parents loved to dance, but somehow sentimental Big Band sounds no longer seemed appropriate. We settled for potluck, conversation, and a cake.

Summer in Leelanau County is a mix of seeing friends who come from the city to enjoy the beauty, and of trying to maintain a work schedule while everyone else seems to be on vacation. Summer of '83 was more of the same, with the difference that we went to see my father, took him for a few outings when he was able, and prepared ourselves emotionally for his death. The grieving process starts early when someone is terminal.

Luckily for us, the nursing home had faces familiar to my father, especially one cousin whom I shall call Meg. When Meg first realized that Dad was coming there, she contemplated quitting her job as an aide, because she thought his presence would be too difficult for her emotionally. Fortunately, she decided to stay and later on was glad she had done so. Still, intimately caring for one's former mentor, now debilitated, was difficult.

My father had been Meg's early elementary teacher. She remembers fondly when she first went to school and he accused her of swearing, because she was speaking Bohemian. She went home, told her father of the incident, who replied, "He wasn't very smart for a teacher." From that day until he could no longer remember Dad had teased her about the incident. He now cooperated at the nursing home more fully with Meg than with the other attendants, she feels, because of their past relationship.

Another aide who worked the night shift was also very kind to my father and used to bring him pudding or applesauce. He always seemed hungry at night when there was no more food available. Perhaps the coolness and texture of these items aided the swallowing of a throat gradually becoming closed. After receiving the nourishment, he would sleep better. Sometimes he would say, "Thank you. That was awfully good."

The night darkness sets a mood different from when there is light to show the way. Most patients are sleeping, but Alzheimer's patients often wake up at any hour and wander through the hallways in search of who knows what. Or perhaps they are wet from urine and want to be dry. Dad would get up occasionally with little or nothing on and walk out of his room. Perhaps, now without a memory, he was looking for something that appeared familiar.

In August I argued my mother's case about her ability to pay the state hospital bill of over $1500 for his ten-day stay there. The hospital's review of her assets had determined that she should be able to pay the entire amount.

My mother and I walked into the antiseptic, institutional hearing room, where three or four people were already seated at a long table. I was reminded of my social work days in Detroit and the bumbling bureaucracy that was sometimes inadvertently created by institutions. The hearings officer briefly stated the name of the case and all the formalities, then inquired as to whether my mother or I wanted to state anything on her behalf. As we had agreed, I responded for her. I felt briefly like an attorney arguing a case. I stated that, even though my mother now had the resources to pay the bill, her assets would quickly dwindle from the eventual payments to nursing homes over an indefinite period. My mother concurred with the argument, and the hearing was over. No one offered any discussion.

The hearings officer stated that our request would be granted and the $1500 would be waived. In fact, all the hearings members acted apologetic, as if they were sorry for the inconvenience of having the hearing in the first place. The judgment was a small victory in the midst of a losing battle, but it buoyed our spirits and made me realize that not all bureaucrats are heartless and cold to the needs of the individual.

Occasionally that summer I took my father for car rides. One time we went to my house to show him our new garage. He didn't show any signs that he recognized me or the house, let alone the new garage. However, to my surprise, he had told me what road to turn down to get to the house and on the return trip showed me how to get to the nursing home. When we arrived at the home, he said, "I better go home now," and it was clear he meant the nursing home.

On a beautiful, sunny, Indian summer day in late October, my mother and I once again took him outside for a walk around the grounds of the home. As we were going out the back door, he noticed a broom standing against the wall. Leaves were scattered on the sidewalk near the door and more were falling from nearby trees. He grabbed the broom as if his assigned task was to sweep leaves off the sidewalk. The activity was the first purposeful task I had seen him perform in many months. My sister told me later that sweeping leaves off the patio decking around the pool was a task he had done in Florida. I watched and waited as he completed the job to his satisfaction. He smiled briefly and we continued our walk. My mother also remembers fondly the day he raked the leaves. However, the activities director's account of his dancing until it "wore her out" was more difficult for Mom to accept. Mom had always loved to dance, but now could not do so because of her healing hip. Oblivious to the dynamics of his actions, my father now danced freely with anyone who would. Whenever the polka band was at the nursing home, he would enthusiastically participate, as he had not done for several years now with Mom. After all his years of controlling, dominating behavior, he finally seemed to let go and become spontaneous. He danced, smiled, and had fun with abandon. But later, he let go in a not so acceptable fashion. He spit on the floor, wet his pants, and wandered from his room *au naturel*. His inhibitions had disappeared.

At Thanksgiving he was still well enough to walk and had adjusted to his home. We brought him home for the holiday meal. Paul and Joanne were home along with her brother Andy, and Jim's 90-year-old grandmother was also on hand. Shortly before mealtime I went to pick up Dad. He looked at his former home as if it belonged to a stranger, but smiled occasionally and as usual was ravenous for food. He sat at the table and ate with us. I had brought a tie from the nursing home to tie him to the chair, as frequently done there, so that he would not get up and wander during the meal. I was reminded of old times when he tried, however inappropriately, to tell a story, and when he ate voraciously at my mother's table. His dominating presence faded, however, as younger personalities took over the limelight.

After dinner I walked with him as he indicated where he wanted to go; to the basement, back upstairs, from room to room to room. Then suddenly he made a motion as if he needed to go to the bathroom. I quickly led him to the toilet seat, but by the time we got there it was too late. Not being accustomed to nursing chores, I nearly got sick when I saw and smelled the feces that soiled his pant leg. He looked at me, shook and lowered his head, and tried to push me away with his hands. His pants were dropped to the floor by now, and shame covered his face. I explained that I knew he was probably embarrassed, but that we needed to change his pants and that I would get the clean pants out of the car that I had brought from the home. I asked Jim to help me keep him in the bathroom while I obtained his clean clothes.

When I returned from the car, Jim was clearly having a hard time keeping him in the bathroom. I talked calmly and soothingly and told him exactly what I was doing. He rubbed his hands on the sides of his pants, looked at me, clucked his tongue, shook his head back and forth, and said, "Dear, dear, dear," as if he were a naughty toddler who had momentarily forgotten his potty training.

Having completed the task of changing his pants, we returned to the activities of the kitchen, which by then had turned to cleaning dishes and putting away food. A stranger in his own house, he looked puzzled as to what his next move should be. It felt good to have him home again, but shortly he was ready to return to what had become his new home. He walked to the door a few times and made it clear that he was ready to leave. Sadly, everyone said, "Goodbye."

I led him outside to the passenger's side of the car. After some confusion as to where he was to enter, he allowed me to help him sit down in the seat. His body was rigid as I swung his legs around to the inside of the car.

Placing the seat belt on him was difficult, as it seemed that his arms were everywhere and he didn't know what to do with them. Exhausted, I drove him back to the nursing home. The time was nearly 7:00 p.m., and the usual activity in and around his room had quieted down. When I returned home, we all commented that the visit had gone as well as it could have and that he had seemed happy to be home for a while. We played a card game and tried to forget.

Christmas that year was quiet. Mother and I took a few gifts to him on Christmas Day, some chocolates that he liked, and a few clothes. He opened the gifts, smiling as if he knew what they were. We thought he knew us that day. By this time the slightest indication of recognition would have been a thrill. I had learned from my mother the ability to experience joy from the little things. I thanked her for that quality now. I felt a kinship with her in our shared pleasure from the touch of a hand or the sweet fragrance from a flower.

In January and February walking became more difficult for my father. His back was hunched over, and he was unable to straighten his legs. Overall he had become weaker, harder to rouse from sleep. When eating in a chair, he would occasionally pitch forward.

Yet, he still smiled once at the end of February when I fed him, as if he were pleased to see me. He still ate whole food then, but in March he had more difficulty and began choking on his food. He had to be fed liquids and would swallow only after being told repeatedly to do so. Then successively large amounts of thick white phlegm would have to be suctioned from his mouth and throat. He had had respiratory problems before, but now the Alzheimer's disease process was most likely the cause of the difficulty.

On Friday, April 6, my Early Music Group came to the nursing home to play for the monthly birthday party. My father couldn't come to the dining room for the music.

He sat in his room, supposedly unaware of his surroundings. Yet as I sang I hoped he could hear me. His room was within earshot. I knew that sensitivity to music remained longer than, say, logical reasoning, and I hoped that on some level the sweet sounds of recorders, lute, and voice reached him and soothed his pain.

That weekend Paul was home to see Dad. On Saturday Dad's muscles were rigid, his mouth was constantly open, he said nothing, and he seemed unaware of anything going on around him. Paul remembers this as the first time our father may not have known he was there. On previous visits Dad had called Paul by name.

Yet a day or two later, less than a week before he died, my mother went with a friend who sang and played the piano for the residents. Mom was sitting with him for over an hour, when he looked at her and said, "Is that you, Viola?" She says, "I'm sure he recognized me then. We wheeled him to his room, and he said, 'Be careful now.'" Those were the last words she heard him speak, for the next time we saw him, the day he died, he spoke only with his eyes.

Chapter XII - Renewal

The tears streamed down my face as fast as the rain poured on the fields around me. I was driving home from a monthly hospice meeting about a year after my father had died. I didn't understand why I was so upset until I thought about what I had done that night. I had volunteered when the nurse had asked for someone to lie in the hospital bed while she demonstrated how to move a dying person in and out of bed. The information she was providing was very helpful to me as a hospice volunteer, because many patients are bedridden for a period of time, and knowing the right body mechanics to use can prevent a back injury.

As the delayed reaction of sadness took over, I realized I had been identifying with my father as he lay in his bed dying. I had tried to simulate dead weight so that the person acting as caretaker would have to use what she had learned to move me. The touch of someone caring for me felt sweet, but the feeling of helplessness, however brief, was overwhelming.

What if I have to go through something like my father did? Every time I walk into a room and temporarily forget what I am looking for, I momentarily wonder if or when I shall become demented. Logic tells me I am being ridiculous, and I move back to the task at hand.

Even now, as I write these words, more than three years after my father's death, I find myself resistant to completing the story, as if when I write the final words I won't be able to hold on to him any longer. Time has been the best healer for the pain of loss, just as the old cliché says, but letting go is still difficult. I stare at the obituary and marvel that a life can be summed up in a few brief paragraphs. I read the autopsy report once again and see the dreaded words "neurofibrillary tangles and neuritic plaques," two key phrases associated with a brain diagnosed as having Alzheimer's.

I remember very little of the funeral except the anti-Semitic comments of the minister and the well intentioned, but insensitive, remarks of a few acquaintances. "He looks just like he did" or "It's a blessing" somehow were not very comforting. What was consoling was the closeness of my mother, brothers, and sister, and the presence of many friends and relatives who remembered my father and related the good times they had had with him.

What helped the most to fill the void was talking about him and his illness and death over and over, and then listening to others' stories and helping them through their pain. My work with the hospice movement in helping dying patients and their families is no accident. My own grieving process is assisted by being around others with similar problems. Death is inevitable, but Alzheimer's disease is not. Someday a cure will be found for this devastation. The ADRDA (Alzheimer's Disease and Related Disorders Association (1-800-621-0379) is trying to make that cure a reality by raising money for research and appropriating it to worthy recipients. The organization has grown a great deal in the past five years and by the end of 1989 had funded more than thirteen million dollars in Alzheimer's research. Realizing that the victim is not the only one who suffers in an Alzheimer's family, the ADRDA also sponsors educational and support programs for families. Many day care facilities are now available, as well as volunteer workers who can provide respite for caregivers.

It is early October now, and the orange and yellow leaves are falling from the trees. Tomorrow's forecast calls for rain possibly mixed with snow. I look out my office window at Sassy, our recently acquired six-month-old quarter horse, and wish my father could be here to see her.

About The Author

Lynn McAndrews has an M.A. in English from Wayne State University in Detroit, Michigan. A former social worker, she has worked with dying patients and their bereaved families. She currently works as a court reporter in northern Michigan and serves as president of the Northwest Michigan Chapter of the Alzheimer's Disease and Related Disorders Association.